MENTAL DISORDER IN THE COMMUNITY
AND IN GENERAL PRACTICE

Mental Disorder in the Community and in General Practice

Doctors' views and patients' demands

PETER F.M. VERHAAK
The Netherlands Institute of Primary Health Care (NIVEL)

Avebury

Aldershot · Brookfield USA · Hong Kong · Singapore · Sydney

Published by
Avebury
Ashgate Publishing Limited
Gower House
Croft Road
Aldershot
Hants GU11 3HR
England

Ashgate Publishing Company
Old Post Road
Brookfield
Vermont 05036
USA

British Library Cataloguing in Publication Data

Verhaak, Peter F.M.
Mental Disorder in the Community and in
General Practice: Doctors' Views and Patients' Demands
I. Title
614.5989009492
ISBN 1-85628-638-X

Library of Congress Catalog Card Number: 94-74549

Printed and bound by Athenaeum Press Ltd.,
Gateshead, Tyne & Wear.

Contents

Preface

This book takes a new look at mental disorder in the population and in primary care settings. The development of theory is based on empirical data, gathered in the Dutch National Survey of Morbidity and Interventions in General Practice. This survey was conducted by NIVEL (the Netherlands Institute of Primary Care) and supported financially by the Ministry of Welfare, Health and Cultural Affairs and the National Health Fund Council.

I would like to thank the following persons for their comments on earlier drafts of this work: Jozien Bensing, Roland Friele, Rob Giel, Peter Groenewegen, Giel Hutschemaekers, Anke de Veer, Jouke van der Zee and my other colleagues from NIVEL.

I would like to thank Marleen Duister and Jan Gravestein for preparation of the data for statistical analysis and Bernadette Kamphuys for her expertise on wordprocessing and lay-out.

Peter F.M. Verhaak

Introduction

So many people are in need of psychiatric treatment (in the view of psychiatrists) and so few are, actually treated. This phenomenon has been discussed frequently, but mostly from a one-sided point of view: the psychiatrist's. Much might be gained by also considering the viewpoints of other parties involved: the patient and the intermediary between patient and psychiatrist, the general practitioner. Hence the subtitle of this book: doctors' views and patients' demands.

It is often difficult for the man in the street to recognize the reality he knows in the state of affairs represented by psychiatric epidemiological figures.

> One or more of the psychiatric disorders ... had been experienced at some time in their lives by 32% of the American adults, and 20% had an active disorder, ...,

Robins, Locke and Regier (1991, p.329) thus begin their concluding chapter on prevalence of psychiatric disorders in America. And such figures are not incidental nor are they a typical product of the latest epidemiological research efforts. In 1964, Taylor and Chave presented a review of studies from 1929 to 1960, giving prevalences of mental disorders, ranging from 0.8% to 81.5% of the population. Leighton, author of one of the studies in this review, wrote:

> we feel fairly sure that 370 per 1000 is the firm core of a prevalence figure for our population; that is, we could expect fairly general agreement among psychiatrists that the individuals represented in the 37 per cent are psychiatric cases and that, whether under treatment or not, they need it (Leighton 1956, p.721).

These high figures are surprising for the layman at first sight. As most of the people consider themselves "normal", they are led to believe that about one in two or three others must be kind of "insane". But, as Michael Shepherd put it in his "Sir Geoffrey Vickers Lecture" of 4 February 1976, we should look beyond the layman's madness to identify the larger part of mental disorder. Shepherd points to the contribution of the so called minor mental disorders (neuroses, personality disorders, behaviour disorders of the childhood, sexual deviation), drug-associated disorders, and mental illness associated with somatic disease, to the prevalences cited above. These minor mental disorders probably form the majority of cases, reported by epidemiologists. The number of psychoses and cases of mental retardation, more easily associated by the layman with psychiatric disorders, are thus reduced to a number, more comprehensible to him. To avoid further misunderstanding, we will use the term "mental disorders" to refer to the whole set of minor mental disorders and the more classical psychiatric disorders together.

Nevertheless, these high figures, about which a lot more can be said, and will be said in the next chapters, are still in contrast to admission rates in mental health services. They don't fit the data about the presentation of mental health problems by patients in primary care either. As will be shown at a later stage, about 5 to 7 per cent of patients, visiting a General Practitioner, bring forward symptoms or complaints of a psychosocial character spontaneously. By "psychosocial", we mean complaints or symptoms referring to emotions, feelings, relationships or material circumstances. The great majority of patients, visiting a General Practitioner, consider their reasons for visit to a doctor physical in nature. And though the General Practitioner may have other reasons as well, relatively few patients are referred to mental health specialists or institutions.

As a result, in the Netherlands 6% of the population above 14 years of age has been treated by a psychiatrist or mental health institution over a 5-year period (Foets and Sixma 1991), although a figure of more than 20% of the population suffering from mental disorder can be reproduced in the Netherlands as well (Hodiamont et al. 1987). In the United States of America, according to the same study which produced a yearly prevalence of 20% of active mental disorders, fewer than one in five persons with such a disorder sought and received care; mental health care being broadly defined to include a single visit to a general medical provider or a mental health specialist for a mental health reason (Klerman et al. 1992).

In short, there is a discrepancy between mental disorder, as defined by psychiatrists and the patients' demands, deduced from requests for help. Of course, it is not a surprising discrepancy. A diagnosis, made by an expert, is based on the symptoms and experience of the patient and cannot be equated with them. One could even argue that that is exactly what experts are for: to shed light on unclear symptoms and to provide a frame of reference to explain the patient's suffering. However, this is where, in case of mental disorder, an intriguing complication comes to the fore. Particularly in case of the minor mental disorders, for which Shepherd demanded attention, the experience of suffering by the patient constitutes an intrinsic aspect of the diagnosis. We are therefore confronted with a situation which can be looked at in three ways: either a lot of people suffer in terms of psychiatric standards, but do not share these standards, or a lot of people suffer but do not seek help, or a lot of people suffer but they are not recognized as suffering. Those sceptical about psychiatric epidemiology (or psychiatry in general) will be inclined to favour the first position arguing that psychiatrists stick the label of illness upon persons with deviant behaviour. Friends and supporters of psychiatry will take the last one, pointing at the incompetence of laymen and generalists to recognize cases of mental disorder. These different positions have been found regularly opposite each other during the last decennia.

The most impressive confrontation between such different positions has been the debate between supporters of social system theories (some of them presenting themselves as "anti-psychiatrists") and those who believed in individual determinants of mental disorder (traditional psychiatrists) in the 60's and early 70's. The anti-psychiatrist stand of Thomas Szasz (1961) may be summarized by the statement that mental illness as such does not exist and that the medical metaphor "illness" was invented in order to suppress potential opponents of the system. Thomas Scheff (1966) argued that reactions of the social environment contribute significantly - along with individual characteristics - to the origin and development of mental disorder. Mental deviation, in his eyes, is a product of a labelling society. Eric Berne (1964), emphasized the interactional element in the process of putting a meaning on someone's behaviour, basing mental disorders on social systems instead of on individual determinants. They all share the idea that people are not so much themselves mentally ill, as made so by society. Psychiatric standards have incorporated society's tendency to normalize, and in fact the need expressed by psychiatric standards is not always felt as such by the individuals who were supposed to suffer. As a result, the demand for help is less than it should be from a psychiatric point of view.

As clinical psychiatrists saw their daily confrontation with suffering people more or less disregarded by "contemporary verbal games", as Shepherd (op.cit., p.91) put it, they reacted furiously against this. As Gerald Klerman, former president of the American Psychiatric Association, said more than twenty years later:

> Psychiatry as a profession had come under attack from anti-psychiatrists, such as Szasz (1961) and Laing (1971); from social scientists, such as the labelling theorists and anthropological relativists; .... The

criticism of psychiatry during the 1960's included more than psychometric issues of validity and reliability, extending to a social and political critique that psychiatry was serving as an agent of social control, disguising its power by benevolent medical rhetoric, imagery and metaphor. Confronted with these widespread and formidable criticisms, the psychiatric research community responded slowly but vigorously (Klerman 1990, p.30).

A more moderate argument occurs at regular intervals when psychiatrists or epidemiologists observe dangerous decreases in community's mental health. Hutschemaekers (1990) traces these observations back to the early eighteenth century, when Cheyne (1671-1743) described the increase of the "English Malady", a kind of hypochondria, to be cured, among other things by returning to the countryside and diets without meat or alcohol. In 1893, Erb (cited by Shorter 1994) spoke of "the growing nervousness of our own age; in 1971 in Dutch medical literature a furious debate was held about the "mental degeneration of the Dutch people". The immediate cause was the inaugural address of Trimbos, professor of Social Psychiatry, who demanded attention for epidemiological data of the kind we mentioned above. His opponent, de Groot, disputed the conclusions drawn by Trimbos, on methodological grounds alone, but the atmosphere in the debate was that of a religious war, between two groups of "believers" (c.f. De Groot 1971, Trimbos 1971).

A last example of the discrepancy between demand for help, put forward by the patient and need, as measured by epidemiologists, arises when the issue of the recognition of mental disorder by general practitioners is raised. Epidemiologists conclude that recognition rates among general practitioners are low:

> Psychiatric interviews (PSE) with patients who were not diagnosed as being mentally disturbed by the General Practitioner in the previous year, indicated mental disturbance in nearly half of the cases (Giel et al. 1991, p.171)[1]

General Practitioners respond by saying:

> there is no reason to presuppose a substantial non-recognition of mental disturbances. On the contrary, General Practitioners recognize or know about most of the cases of mental disturbance. If they do not pay attention to them, they have there reasons for it in most cases... The fact that, ... people with psychological problems "run wild" is

1 Originally Dutch citation, translated by PV

> another story. It is debatable whether these people should be detected and sneaked into the medical circuit. And the conclusion of the debate does not impose a prior requirement for the General Practitioner to detect them (Van der Velden 1991, in a commentary with Giel et al., p.155).

Goldberg commented on such situations twenty years ago saying that

> in a case, detected by a psychiatric screening test the patient ... (will) typically be aware of her symptoms but will either consider herself not ill at all or physically ill (Goldberg 1974, p.1245).

As was said before, this discrepancy between the need established among the population in terms of psychiatric norms and the demand for help is an intriguing one and worth studying further. Questions that need to be answered include the following: What is the subjective experience of those who are classified as disturbed by psychiatry? For what reason do they not arrive at the gates to psychiatric help? Who seeks help and who does not? And, how do patients manage, who should be in treatment according to Leighton's citation on page 1, but who actually are not? These answers should not be given in the terminology of psychiatry alone. Thanks to numerous psychiatric epidemiological investigations, we already know a lot about mental disorder as psychiatrists[1] define it; but too little about mental disorder as patients experience it. Knowledge about mental disorder as psychiatrists define it is knowledge of "diseases". Where disorder is a category like "illness", patient's experience of being ill, "disease" is a derivative of it, a scientific abstraction. A disease is a kind of external state by which patients are affected. Disease can be diagnosed by experts, on the basis of objective definitions. Knowledge about disease is necessary but not sufficient to provide an understanding of the epidemiology of human suffering and problem solving. Such an understanding has to take into account the subjective experience of being mentally unwell and its relationship with disease as well.

Moreover, solely relying on knowledge about disease might be misleading too. Classification in terms of "diseases" gives the "disease" approach a monopoly:

> if you can't label it, you can't count it; if you can't count it, it does not exist an therefore it is not worth labeling,

White (1988, p.41) ironically observes. As long as the complex concept of mental disorder is only described in the reductionist terminology of scientific disease classification, such a reduction will represent "reality". Whether this representation is suitable depends on the questions one wishes to answer. This representation might be very useful indeed to describe a population in an objective way, or to provide a common language for the sake of communication between providers. For the purpose of out-reach offering unrequested help or mental health care planning, other viewpoints (especially the patient's) should be taken into consideration. Therefore, it is crucial to at least try to describe the subjective point of view of the patient as well.

And here we arrive at the main goal of this book. This is, to combine the interpretation of disease and the subjective experience of patients, in order to obtain an integrated picture of the doctor's view and patient's requirements. The data which provide this picture were gathered during a nationwide survey of Morbidity and Interventions in General Practice, carried out by the Netherlands Institute of Primary Care in 1987-1988. For the purposes of this study, all doctor-patient contacts in a population of 335,000 patients in 103 Dutch general practices were recorded during a three month period. A random sample of about 16,000 patients from this population was extensively interviewed. The combination of both data-sets provides us with information about feelings of distress, experienced by patients, problem situations, and indicators of mental illness and also about their help-seeking behaviour during the three months, the complaints they presented to their General Practitioners, diagnoses made by the General Practitioner and consequently, treatment or possible referral.

This data presents the opportunity of analyzing mental disorder in the community, help seeking behaviour as a consequence of such disorder, the resulting morbidity presented in general practice and general practitioners' treatment of such complaints. The whole pathway to a possible psychiatric diagnosis will be studied from the perspective of psychiatric epidemiologists, of general practitioners and of the patients themselves.

The book is organized as follows:

Chapter 1 presents a further theoretical elaboration of the problem sketched above. How is mental disorder defined, how can it be measured and what is the tension between doctor's views and patient's demands.

Chapter 2 summarizes research method and instruments, used in the National Survey, mentioned above. This chapter is of a somewhat academic nature, which is considered necessary to enable the reader to estimate the results at their true value. It contains information about the representative nature of the data and about the instruments used.

Chapter 3 describes psychiatric morbidity in the population, as it is experienced by the patient and as it is defined by psychiatrists. Chapter 3 also discusses the patient's decision to seek help. In this chapter the issue raised at the beginning of the chapter, i.e. the large number of cases of mental disorder in the population, according to psychiatrists without appropriate treatment is the central point.

Chapter 4 is dedicated to the complaints presented to the general practitioner and the recognition of mental disorder by the General Practitioner. Special attention is paid to the demands for help from those subgroups of patients who either report experience of mental distress themselves (and thus are in subjective need) or via psychiatric screening-questionnaires (objective need).

Chapter 5 describes treatment by the General Practitioner. It is relevant in several ways: it is important to assess how patients are treated in case of mental disorder, which may be a disorder in the view of the professional without any experience of distress by the patient, or an experience of distress without a probable disorder in psychiatric eyes, or a disorder on which everybody agrees. It is also important to assess what patient characteristics determine the likelihood of treatment. One aspect of the General Practitioner's treatment, his capacity to refer the patient to a more specialized agency, brings us to the end of the scope of our work.

Chapter 6 discusses the consequences of this study for the picture of mental illness in the community and in general practice.

Notes

1. The terms "psychiatrist" and "psychiatric" viewpoints are oversimplifications, referring to the naturalistic paradigm in psychiatry (cf. Wulff, Pederson and Rosenberg, 1986), being the current vision in the last decades.

1 Theoretical considerations

The gentle art of making simple things complicated

In the introductory chapter the research problem was presented as the contrast between psychiatric epidemiological data and patients' demands for psychiatric help. In this chapter we will elaborate - and also complicate - this contrast.

From a historical point of view, one should realize that the first professional descriptions of mental disorder stem from the mental hospital. When in the first half of the twentieth century psychiatric epidemiologists began to describe psychiatric morbidity outside the asylum, the nomenclature developed in institutional settings was exported to the community. However, definitions that are applicable to an institutionalized population cannot automatically be applied to persons in the population at large. The ideal types encountered in the mental hospital do not present themselves as such in the population.

When we discuss the difference between the patient's perspective and the psychiatrist's the general practitioner plays an intermediary role. At first, most patients arrive at primary care settings with an unordered set of complaints and symptoms. The general practitioner selects some of them for psychiatric referral and keeps many for treatment in primary care. Primary care physicians are seldom confronted with the clear-cut cases they have been taught about during their training in psychiatric wards. On the contrary, they run across patients with vague symptoms, perhaps borderline cases, on whom psychiatric diagnoses seldom apply. For this reason, general practitioners have developed their own concepts and classification schemes, where more room is reserved for symptomatology.

When we define mental disorder in this chapter, we will consider the definition in two contexts. We will first define mental disorder according to the frame of reference of the psychiatrist, then the general practitioner and finally the patient. Secondly, we will consider mental disorder at different levels in the health care system: in the population, in primary care and within specialized mental health care settings.

Before starting this definition exercise, one etymological remark needs to be made. We refer to "mental disorder" as the concept we are defining. When we are defining it from the perspective of the medical model, we might refer to "mental illness", "mental disease" or "psychiatric disease" respectively "diagnosis". In these cases, a (medical) diagnosis has been made. The diagnosis was based on the symptoms, presented by the patient. When we refer to the way a patient experiences feelings of being emotionally or psychologically unwell, we use concepts like "psychological", "emotional" or "psychosocial" problems / symptoms / complaints. The difference between problems and complaints on the one hand and symptoms on the other is the clinical relevance of the latter. A symptom is considered as an indicator for a medical diagnosis by the clinician (c.f. Koeter 1992).

Mental disorder according to psychiatrists:

The psychiatric disease concept

Psychiatry is traditionally a medical discipline and mental disorders are thus considered in that context as "diseases". At least, this has been the situation since about half of the former century. Ideally, a disease is an entity that can be objectively defined by its etiology (most preferable), pathogenesis or symptoms. Especially when the etiology, and thus the cause of disease is known, a doctor can predict its course and take decisions regarding the most desirable therapy. This situation, which made physical medicine so successful in case of infectious diseases, makes the disease model desirable for psychiatric illnesses too. There is a problem, however. Let us take for example influenza. Doctors can agree on criteria as to when a person is to be defined a "flu patient". It is true that some of the patients in question may not feel at all "fluey" (and there may well be others who would like to qualify as "flu patients", but do not), but in this case there are objective biochemical criteria that can be taken to indicate the presence or absence of the flu virus.

One of the features of most mental disorders is the very lack of this kind of physical substratum which enables one to decide unambiguously whether or not a patient is suffering from such a disorder. This situation may change in due course, but anno 1994 psychiatrists and other clinicians have to rely on agreement among themselves on the criteria they apply to the predicate "disturbed" in respect of particular behaviour, feelings or requests for help. As we shall see below, the current way of categorizing mental disorder relies heavily on such agreements.

The "disease interpretation" has two important features. First, it is the expert, the doctor, who determines the diagnosis. Disease is an entity distinct from the patient. By analogy with physical diseases, mental disorder is regarded as a condition that can be unambiguously defined on the basis of its symptoms and course. This interpretation is important for the clinician as well as for the epidemiologist. It provides a basis for treatment and for communication between professionals (for example the referring general practitioner and the psychiatrist consulted). This last aspect, the common language, is especially important for the epidemiology: if we are to arrive at a reliable classification of disorders, we desperately need such a definition. And a reliable classification is the first necessary condition in order to be able to count and provide a good epidemiological overview.

The second feature of the "disease interpretation" is the conceptualization of mental disorders as entities, as distinct categories which can clearly be distinguished from one another. This is a more debatable point, even among psychiatrists.

In an introductory editorial in Psychological Medicine, Häfner (1987) wrote,

> Development of disease constructs for certain mental disorders is meaningful if they provide at least an adequate explanation of the symptom clusters, the underlying pathological mechanisms and the course of the disorder. (Häfner 1987, p.14)

But in his view disorders that are better explained as learned behaviour ought not to be described as "diseases". So, a disease construct for Alzheimer's disease or major depression, is more acceptable in his eyes than a similar definition for agoraphobia. In general, classical psychiatric syndromes are well suited to a definition in terms of disease.

In the same spirit, Wulff, Pederson and Rosenberg (1986) conclude that

> it remains a fact at present the biological disease concept is better founded in psychotic conditions than in neuroses and personality disorders. Most psychiatrists agree that psychoses are diseases in a medical sense (Wulff, Pederson and Rosenberg 1986, p.112)

These disorders are encountered relatively infrequently in the community and in general practice, but often in psychiatric hospitals.

However, if we consider those mental disorders that occur more frequently, it seems hardly justified to consider them as entities and to try and classify them in mutually exclusive categories. The metaphor of the medical model resulting in mental disease categories such as anxiety or depression has been severely criticized, for instance by psychologists such as Eysenck. In the words of the latter:

> Diagnostic categories .... are a scientific anachronism, but professional consensus among psychiatrists and their need to justify themselves to other physicians as practising a proper medical specialty treating categorical disease entities demand categories (Eysenck, Wakefield and Friedman 1983, p.185).

The reason for diagnostic categories in psychiatry being scientifically unsound in general has been expressed by Kraüpl Taylor (1971). Put briefly, Kraüpl Taylor's criticism is as follows:

- Psychiatric categories are not logically mutually exclusive;
- The same syndrome may have several causes, and one cause may result in various syndromes;
- Psychiatric illness is treated as being a matter of all or nothing, whereas the transitions are generally gradual;
- Characteristics in terms of dimensions are regarded as separate entities.

As we shall see below, the current classification systems in psychiatric epidemiology (the Diagnostic Statistical Manual, DSM, of which the fourth version has appeared) are categorical systems (although mutual exclusion of categories is not required in the strictest sense, because patients are allowed to suffer from several diseases). Thus, Eysenck et al., offering recommendations for future revisions of the psychiatric classification system DSM-III, propose first to replace categorical diagnosis with dimensional assessment.

In this connection Goldberg and Huxley (1992) discuss the common mental disorders "anxiety" and "depression" and the difficulty of distinguishing them from one other as separate categories. This proves impossible for a variety of reasons:

- The more anxious people become, the more depressive they become, and vice versa: these are not exclusive categories;
- People who score high on "anxiety" and those who score high on "depression" turn out to have the same sociodemographic characteristics and the same co-morbidity;
- In both cases the transition between the category of illness and that of normality is a gradual one;
- The reliability with which patients can be classified in one category or the other is limited;
- The stability of a diagnosis over a period of time is limited;
- Effects of treatment are independent of the diagnosis.

Based on the factual material they present (see also the overview by Angst

1990), Goldberg and Huxley suggest a dimensional model for "common mental disorders". They base this on an "anxiety dimension" and a "depression dimension". A number of symptoms are indicative on both axes. However, there is a certain line along each dimension above which psychopathology can be said to exist. How many symptoms are allowed before deciding that a disorder exists remains arbitrary.

Foulds (1976) points to the same phenomenon that various disorders tend to go together, and as such mitigate against a classification of "illnesses" in categories. He postulates a hierarchy of mental disorders and, on the basis of empirical research, distinguishes four levels of disorder which form a cumulative scale. If a person is suffering from a disorder at the highest level, he will generally also be suffering from disorders at the levels below. The levels distinguished by Foulds are:

1) non-integrated psychotics, patients with a distorted picture of reality, which cannot be controlled.
2) integrated psychotics, whose disturbed picture of the world can be kept under control by means of medication.
3) neurotics
4) people suffering from mood disturbances.

The hierarchy worked for 93 per cent of the 480 persons examined in a psychiatric clinic; in other words, where the diagnosis was "neurosis" or "integrated psychosis", the patient was also suffering from mood disturbances, but not vice versa. Thirteen per cent were not suffering from any disorder at all, 18 per cent were only suffering from a mood disturbance, 34 per cent showed neurotic symptoms (and mood disturbances), 19 per cent were suffering from delusions which could be kept under control (and neurotic symptoms and mood disturbances) and 8 per cent from non-integrated psychoses.

According to this theory, less serious disorders are always found in people with serious mental disorders, without being specific to the serious disorder in question. In a large-scale study in the Netherlands at the beginning of the eighties, (Hodiamont, Peer and Syben 1987) the extent to which a population of 3000 persons had a psychiatric disease and the extent to which they were experiencing psychosocial problems was established. Most of the psychiatric cases in the project also experienced psychosocial problems, while, conversely, most of the patients with psychosocial problems (of whom there were many more than the psychiatric cases) did not have psychiatric problems (Hodiamont 1986). The danger Hodiamont points out is that for many patients, where the two kinds of problem occur simultaneously, the psychosocial problems ("which we all have at some time or another") mask the more serious psychiatric problems. The other side of this is that names are used for the psychosocial problems that are derived from "full-blown psychiatry", and thus create the opposite confusion.

The similarity between these findings and those of Foulds' will be clear. Most people with serious psychiatric problems are also in great personal distress, but not everybody who experiences emotional distress has a serious psychiatric problem.

We have dwelled for some time on the topic of mental disorder as a category or dimension because of its implications for disorders encountered at the population and primary care level. It should be emphasized that in current research practice, the disease concept is not affected by a dimensional interpretation of mental disorder. This is because, within that dimensional interpretation it remains possible, and is in fact customary, to draw demarcation lines and divide the world into two categories: those scoring above and those scoring below these lines.

Thus, in current psychiatric research practice people are categorized as mentally ill according to objective criteria, irrespective of the patient's own evaluation of his condition.

Measurement of mental disorder in psychiatric epidemiology

A classification of "mental disorders" as separate entities is extremely useful, especially for epidemiological purposes. Epidemiology is, among other things, a matter of counting and countable units are a prerequisite for counting.

Originally, the point of departure was the psychiatric nosology as formulated by Kraepelin. The classical syndromes, mostly psychotic disorders like dementia praecox, dementia, affective psychoses and manic-depressive disorders were classified in the International Classification of Diseases (ICD). Less severe disturbances, the neurotic disorders, constituted kind of a residual category. One of the major problems with these disease-categories was the far from complete agreement between different diagnosticians. Mcguire (1973) provides an overview of reliability research, indicating average over-all agreement scores between 32% and 63%[1].

Dohrenwend (1990) briefly sketches the history of psychiatric epidemiological research. Such an enterprise had, until 1940, to rely on ICD-diagnoses, made by clinicians who got their information often from informants. Cases were counted on the basis of informants' reports, prevalence and incidence were equivalent to the number of cases known to psychiatrists and the number of new referrals respectively.

In the second generation of epidemiological studies (1940-1970), which includes several classic studies such as the Midtown Manhattan Study and the Stirling County Study, some degree of standardization exists. Psychiatrists conducted clinical interviews with a sample of the population; more or less standardized interviews were used, which were sometimes even struc-

tured in such a way as to produce standard scores (for example the Langner Scale). These American studies did not state their outcomes in the form of detailed diagnostic categories (as was the tradition in Europe), but rather confined themselves to the dichotomy between case and non-case (Klerman 1990). The major imperfections of this situation remained the
"little consensus ... about the population of signs and symptoms to be sampled", as Dohrenwend (p.197) puts it, and the lack of criterion-oriented validity. The first comment points to the lack of a common nomenclature to replace the old ICD-categories, that were found not suitable anymore. The latter comment indicates the lack of any

> attempt to test the ability of the diagnostic procedure to identify and classify known cases of important types or to test whether the main measures agreed with very different measures of the same types of disorders (Dohrenwend, p.197).

Since 1970, important developments have taken place, that should at least solve the problem of lack of common nomenclature and standardization. Three major innovations deserve our attention.

1) **DSM-III.** This is the third revised version of the Diagnostic Statistical Manual. DSM-III gives precise operational definitions, which must be satisfied before a patient is put into a particular diagnostic category. It claims to establish psychopathology in an objective and reliable fashion, using standardized interviews in which the history of the illness and the symptoms are recorded. Objective, because the outcome is independent of the preoccupations of the person making the diagnosis. Reliable, because the definitions are so unambiguous that, in principle, every evaluator should reach the same conclusion. In DSM-III, disorders are classified according to explicit inclusion and exclusion criteria, yielding disorders that are either shown or presumed to be distinguished by other differences in course of illness, familial pattern, and predisposing factors (APA, 1980). DSM-III is a-theoretical in nature. The various diagnostic categories are descriptive and do not imply an etiological basis in the disorders. The nonetiological, atheoretical, and descriptive nature of the DSM-III was intentional so as not to alienate potential users from diverse theoretical orientations (Eysenck, Wakefield and Friedman 1983). DSM-III provided psychiatry with a common language, precisely because it eschews a theoretical basis.

2) **Screening instruments.** A second development is the further elaboration of screening questionnaires, already started with the introduction of the Langner-22 scale. Because of its relatively low prevalence,

screening large samples of the population for the existence of psychopathology was a time-consuming exercise. This is why questionnaires were developed that could be administered quickly, and whose outcomes showed a high degree of correspondence with the presence of psychopathology. It thus became possible to screen large groups of the population, using the General Health Questionnaire (GHQ), (Goldberg 1972), the Symptom Check List (SCL-90) (Derogatis 1977, Arindell and Ettema 1986), the Centre of Epidemiological Studies Depression Scale (CES-D), (Radloff 1977) or the Psychiatric Epidemiological Research Interview (PERI), (Shrout, Dohrenwend and Levav 1986). In general, a score above a given threshold indicates that there is an increased likelihood of psychopathology. Thresholds are chosen in such a way that a maximal number of "true cases" are identified while a minimal number of "non-cases" are wrongly indicated as a case. Some of the instruments (SCL-90, PERI) provide scores on several dimensions (for instance depression, anxiety, or somatization) while the original form of the GHQ limits itself to an over-all score. After a first screening with a screening-instrument a standardized interview is conducted to arrive at DSM-diagnoses with the group of potential "cases", as well as with a small proportion of the remainder. In this way a relatively expensive method of data collection can be employed in a comparatively economical fashion.

3) **PSE and DIS.** To provide a standardized approach to DSM-III diagnoses, a number of standardized clinical interview schedules have been developed. The Present State Examination and the Diagnostic Interview Schedule are the most often used standardized interviews for establishing psychopathology in the manner outlined above. DIS results directly in DSM-III diagnoses, PSE, though in fact developed before DSM-III, has a similar function.

Psychiatric classification has thus become more objectified than ever. There is a division into categories: either a person is a case or he is not, and if he is a case there is a name for the disease, and all this according to standards that are outside the patient's control. Klerman (1990) regards DSM-III as a victory for the neo-Kraepelinians.

> The essential tenet of this Neo-Kraepelinian paradigm was that psychiatry was the specialty of medicine...The categorical approach to mental illness emphasized the theory and measurement of these disorders (Klerman 1990, p.29).

In his view it is now time to get back to "normal science" and pluck the rewards: the reliability and validity of screening instruments must be improved; as validation improves so will knowledge about etiology and pathophysiology; a good insight into the incidence of various psychiatric diseases will be developed by means of longitudinal studies; and when the diseases can finally be properly established it will be time for international and cross-cultural comparisons and comparisons over time.

Have these developments resolved the problems of inadequate nomenclature and lack of validity?

DSM-III anyhow has introduced a common nomenclature. Since 1980 it has become customary in clinical practice as well as in epidemiological research to refer to DSM-III categories. Eysenck, Wakefield and Friedman (1983) in their rather critical discussion of DSM-III (see above) report more satisfactory agreements than was the case in earlier research. Over-all kappa's range from .66-.78, kappa being a more severe criterium than the earlier percentages agreement, reported by McGuire (1973).

More comments have been made, however, regarding the way one should arrive at DSM-III diagnoses: the standardized interviews and screening questionnaires. Dohrenwend (1990) remarks that little research has been done into the validity of semi-structured interviews. These measuring instruments derive their credibility from the fact that they were developed on the basis of psychiatric cases, and this is considered a weak basis for use in the community at large. This is demonstrated by conducting one of these semi-structured interviews (the Psychiatric Status Schedule) with samples of the population and with psychiatric patients. The internal consistency of the various scales proved good when applied to the latter group, but not at all so within the cross-section sample. In that group PSS grossly overestimated the occurrence of a diagnosis such as "schizophrenia", when compared to the diagnosis reached by a psychiatrist in an independent interview. Dohrenwend does not regard this result as applying specifically to PSS, but to any standardized interview modeled on a psychiatric population.

Similar results emerge from research into another interview schedule, the PSE by Wing et al. (1978). Only one of the 22 women from a sample of the general population that the PSE indicated as having a "depressive disorder" satisfied the "Feighner Criteria" (a clinical standard). Of a sample of in-patients in a psychiatric hospital, 16 of the 23 selected by the test satisfied the criteria.

A different kind of problem is noted by Dohrenwend, following validation studies on the Diagnostic Interview Schedule. The diagnoses obtained by psychiatrists using the DIS correspond reasonably well with the results of their own assessment, but the degree of correspondence is much less when a DIS diagnosis reached by a lay interviewer is compared with that of a psychiatrist. This low degree of correspondence is dramatically illustrated when DIS lifetime diagnoses (assessed by lay interviewers) are compared with lifetime diagnoses of the same patients one year later: 2456 out of 3572 cases with a lifetime diagnosis for a particular disorder did not have a lifetime diagnosis one year later (Dohrenwend 1990, p.203). Here, reliability of the lay interviewer as well as reliability of the answers obtained with a self report method are under discussion.

The screening questionnaires, such as the GHQ, also suffer validity problems. According to Dohrenwend, their correlation with factors such as self-esteem, helplessness/hopelessness, grief and confusion is extremely high. We came across this phenomenon in our own research, when we tried to correlate GHQ scores of patients who had sought help from social work agencies with the presence of psychopathology, measured using DIS (Friele and Verhaak 1991). We found no connection between the two measures, which must probably be attributed to the extreme hopelessness and grief experienced by the respondents at the time, which resulted in high GHQ scores in all cases. The expected relationship was clearly demonstrable within an out-patient mental health population, which was probably selected more on the basis of psychopathology as the primary cause of the trouble (Friele and Verhaak 1991).

Nevertheless, broadly speaking this is the situation on the basis of which current figures, as presented in the Introduction, are produced. These are figures from the psychiatric point of view. Methodologically speaking, they are better than the figures presented thirty years ago. They are based on generally accepted and widely used operational definitions, which means that morbidity figures have become much easier to compare. There is more general agreement as to when a person is suffering from a "psychiatric illness". On the other hand, as we have demonstrated on the foregoing pages, there are serious methodological shortcomings.

Even if these shortcomings are taken away, we should bear in mind that those figures are based on one specific frame of reference, the medical disease model. The unanimity reached is based on arbitrary agreements about the number of symptoms required to be able to say something is a "definite case" of a particular category, as in DSM-III or PSE, or about the cut-off points applied in the screening instruments, such as GHQ.

What is more, it would seem that these standardized methods are more specific when used on a preselected population than when they are applied to the population at large. This is a point for discussion in the section of this chapter on the different levels where mental disorder can be measured. First we will look at the concept of mental disorder from the view of general practitioners and patients.

Mental disorder from the viewpoint of general practitioners

Diagnoses in primary care settings

Lamberts (1991) has introduced a taxonomy of diagnoses in general practice, which may clarify the differences between morbidity in general practice and morbidity in specialist settings. A medical diagnosis, reflecting by definition the evaluation by a doctor of the request for help by the patient in medical terms, may be based on evidence of pathological-anatomical or pathophysiological nature. These diagnoses are labelled as *pathological* or *pathophysiological* diagnoses which refer definitely at diseases, and which can be concluded to on basis of objective evidence.

A next category Lamberts distinguishes is the *nosological* diagnosis. The etiology and pathological or pathophysiological substratum are unknown. They are a result of consensus between doctors to define certain combinations of symptoms as an illness. The family of psychiatric illnesses, discussed previously, belongs largely to this category.

As we defined earlier, symptoms are complaints, brought forward by the patient, which are indicators for medical diagnoses, be they pathological, pathophysiological or nosological diagnoses. A symptom, such as headache, might refer to a whole number of different diagnoses. However, the diagnosis of the general practitioner often remains limited to such a symptom: i.e. "*symptom-diagnosis*".

Finally, general practice is confronted with requests for help concerning psychological or social problems which cannot be defined as "illness", not even on nosological grounds. These are problems which, though not considered illnesses, require medical help and for which the general practitioner feels responsible. Examples of such problems are nervousness, relational problems or working problems and they are labelled by Lamberts as "*problem behaviour*". A more or less comparable category is that of "*functional complaints*" :physical sensations resulting from emotions, for which no pathological or pathophysiological explanation can be found. Again, it is legitimate to seek medical help and general practitioners consider treatment their business. Whereas pathological and pathophysiological diagnoses can be established objectively; problem behaviour and functional complaints exist only because help was sought for them.

A feature of morbidity in general practice is that general practitioners come across relatively few "ideal types" of syndromes and many more cases of individual symptoms, or even more subjectively, problem behaviour and functional complaints. Specialists work with patients who have illnesses that are both more severe and less likely to remit spontaneously than those commonly seen by family doctors (Goldberg 1992). As we shall discuss in greater detail below, it is precisely for this reason that primary care morbidity classifications suitable for the registration of symptom-diagnoses as well as fully elaborated medical diagnoses, have been developed. Lamberts (1991), using such a primary care oriented classification system (the International Classification for Primary Care: ICPC) demonstrated the overrepresentation of "symptom-diagnoses" for the psychosocial domain as well as for physical illnesses. His results show that if one considers the initial contacts in an episode of illness - and 80 per cent of episodes of illness consist of no more than one contact - over 80 per cent of the diagnoses in which mental disturbance or social problems are found, consists of symptom diagnoses. However, also in the sections "Musculoskeletal", "Neurological" and "Female Genital System", half or more of the initial contacts are diagnosed on the basis of symptoms.

The situation is of course different in follow-up contacts within a single episode of illness. In follow-up contacts the general practitioner has had opportunities to carry out further diagnostics and as time goes by, more understanding is gained in the course of the illness. Nevertheless, even after follow-up contacts, diagnoses based on symptoms still comprise 60 per cent of diagnoses where mental disturbance is found; 100 per cent where the diagnosis is social problems; 75 per cent of diagnoses within the "Female Genital System"; and more than 20 per cent in such common areas as "General", "Digestive", "Musculoskeletal", "Neurological", "Respiratory" and "Pregnancy". In other words, "symptom diagnosis" is very common in general practice.

Compared with the psychiatric disease concept, as elaborated earlier in this chapter, the viewpoint of the general practitioner leaves more room for the experiences and perceptions of the patient. In doing so, he is able to incorporate the context in which the symptoms occur. Symptoms are not simply considered as contributing to an "objective" classification or diagnosis, but viewed within the situation in which they appear. Concepts like "problem behaviour" and "functional complaints" provide the general practitioner with the opportunity to take the context into account.

Classification in general practice

Current morbidity classifications in general practice reflect these characteristics of morbidity in general practice. Compared to a specialist, a general practitioner sees relatively few well-defined syndromes and relatively large numbers of symptoms for which it is (as yet) impossible to give a definite diagnosis. Of the approximately 9,000 ailments in the International Classification of Diseases (ICD), general practitioners come across some 1,000 with some regularity (Lamberts 1991). That means that general practitioners have always had a need for classifications that are on the one hand limited to those disorders that can be regularly expected in primary care, while at the same time enabling them to respond to symptoms and so-called ill-defined conditions.

The oldest classification for general practitioners, the E-list, is basically an extract from the ICD. The first classification that was developed specially for general practitioners was the International Classification of Health Problems in Primary Care (ICHPPC), which was an attempt to meet the needs of general practitioners as outlined above while still retaining a link with the ICD. Mental disorders are classified in broad diagnostic terms, derived from the psychiatric categories within the ICD. However, it also has a typically general practice section containing social and family problems. It cannot be used to classify the patient's complaint. This was felt to be an omission (Lamberts 1982).

This was why the International Classification of Primary Care (ICPC) was developed, in which the Reason for Encounter was adopted as the starting point (c.f. Lamberts and Wood 1987; Lamberts, Meads and Wood 1982). The reason a patient consults a general practitioner may be because he is experiencing symptoms or complaints, or it may be because of a previous diagnosis. This is why, for each section (which include Psychological and Social, in addition to, for example, Digestive, Eye, Skin and Male Genital System) the ICPC has a sub-section of symptoms and a sub-section of diagnoses. The latter have more or less been imported from ICHPPC-II. In addition, each section contains categories in which to record a patient's request for a medicine, an examination, or a referral. In other words the ICPC to some extent reflects the general practitioner's focus on what the patient wants.

The ICPC may be used to classify the reasons for encounter presented by the patient, but also to classify the diagnosis of the general practitioner. This means that a general practitioner not only may use psychiatric diagnoses for the classification of mental problems, but is also able to confine himself to emotional symptoms, such as feeling nervous or depressed. The reason for the consultation can also be classified in terms of a wide range of relational, family and material problems, and each "physical" section also contains help-seeking behaviour that is connected with the fear of a particular illness or the mental and emotional problems such a complaint can cause.

The problems of reliability which hampered psychiatry before the arrival of standardized classifications apply all the more to classifications in primary care, with its global and poorly defined categories. Jenkins, Smeeton and Shepherd (1988) carried out research into the manner in which general practitioners classified emotional disorders using two systems of classification, ICD and ICHPPC-II. They conclude that general practitioners rarely agree among themselves as to the diagnoses they make, that often no diagnosis is made at all, that they agree better as to the individual psychological, somatic and social features (symptoms) than to the resulting diagnosis, and that they often feel that all three components are involved at the same time. Nevertheless, despite the defects in the systems of classification they examined, the authors feel that the value of classification as such is not denied, because, as they put it, "to discard classification is to discard scientific thinking". Field studies and feasibility studies have been conducted for the ICPC, but neither reliability nor inter-doctor variation has been studied systematically.

The patient's view

Regarding the patient's definition of his situation, his subjective needs as we may call them, we can be rather short. To begin with, the patient has sensations. Sensations which are pleasant or unpleasant. Sensations which sometimes have a significant meaning for the patient, implying that help-seeking is desirable, legitimate or perhaps even necessary. In such cases, sensations become problems. These evaluations may be different for each patient, dependent on his health beliefs, his layman's vision and the extent to which he has been initiated into mental health affairs. Some problems result in complaints for which a medical solution seems desirable and there is a demand for help. As we mentioned earlier, when professionals are confronted with such demands, they recognize complaints as symptoms, possibly implying a diagnosis. At that moment the translation from demand to a need in the eyes of a professional has been made. More will be said about this in the following section.

What needs to be noted about the patient's view yet, is its ego-syntomic character. A patient's experience of psychological problems is solely dependent on his own experience. One cannot measure psychological problems in a patient who himself is not aware of them, in contradistinction to some diagnoses of "mental illness" which are to be made by professionals without agreement of the patient, as we saw earlier.

Classifications of patient's own subjective feelings are numerous. They vary from answers on questions "how have you been feeling in general?" to detailed questionnaires such as the Nottingham Health Profile (Hunt et al., 1986)) or the Sickness Impact Profile (Deyo et al., 1983). But in fact, answers on screening questionnaires or psychiatric interviews may be considered reports of patient's subjective feelings too, if one limits oneself to the answers sec. At the moment that answers are combined or added together on theoretical grounds and cut-off points are calculated, the subjective feeling ends and the professional frame of reference is introduced.

Mental disorder at several levels within the health care system

It has been mentioned several times before, that mental disorder can be observed at various levels within the health care system and that the level of observation has consequences for the content validity of the diagnoses made. The validity and reliability of psychiatric classification tends to decrease as the population examined becomes less selected (Dohrenwend 1990). The population is of course least selected at the level of the community at large, before any demand for help has been developed. It becomes more selected when we consider the patients visiting primary care workers, usually general practitioners or primary care physicians while the most selected level is that where patients are admitted to a mental hospital.

These different levels come back in what is known as Goldberg and Huxley's model (Goldberg and Huxley 1980, 1992). Goldberg and Huxley distinguished between five levels at which mental disorders could manifest themselves, five levels among which there are filters that have to be passed in order to progress from one level to the next. In consequence, in an "ideal type" of case, at each subsequent level there are fewer "cases" than at the previous one. Figure 1.1 illustrates Goldberg and Huxley's model.

At the first level, the incidence of mental disorders in the population is considered. Level II contains all those people with mental disorders who have been seen in primary care. Thus we can say that the first filter to be passed is the decision to manifest "illness behaviour". As Mechanic (1986) puts it,

> Illness behaviour involves the manner in which individuals monitor their bodies, define and interpret their symptoms and symptom change over the course of an illness and how this affects behaviour, the remedial actions taken, and response to treatment. (Mechanic 1986, p.1)

In other words, a simple visit to the doctor stands for a world of considerations and decisions. After level II there is another filter: the general practitioner has to recognize that the patient has a mental illness. As a result, level III includes all those people with mental disorders who have consulted a general practitioner and whose problems have been designated mental illness by him. The next filter is the general practitioner's decision to refer the patient to a more specialized mental health agency. If he does not do this, but decides to treat the problem himself (by talking to the patient, prescribing antidepressants or hoping that time will bring a cure) the patient remains at the third level. However, if he does refer the patient, the patient reaches level IV, psychiatric care. And if, ultimately, the final filter is passed and it is decided to admit the patient to a psychiatric hospital, he has reached level V. In Goldberg and Huxley's terminology the patient has completed his "Pathway to psychiatric care".

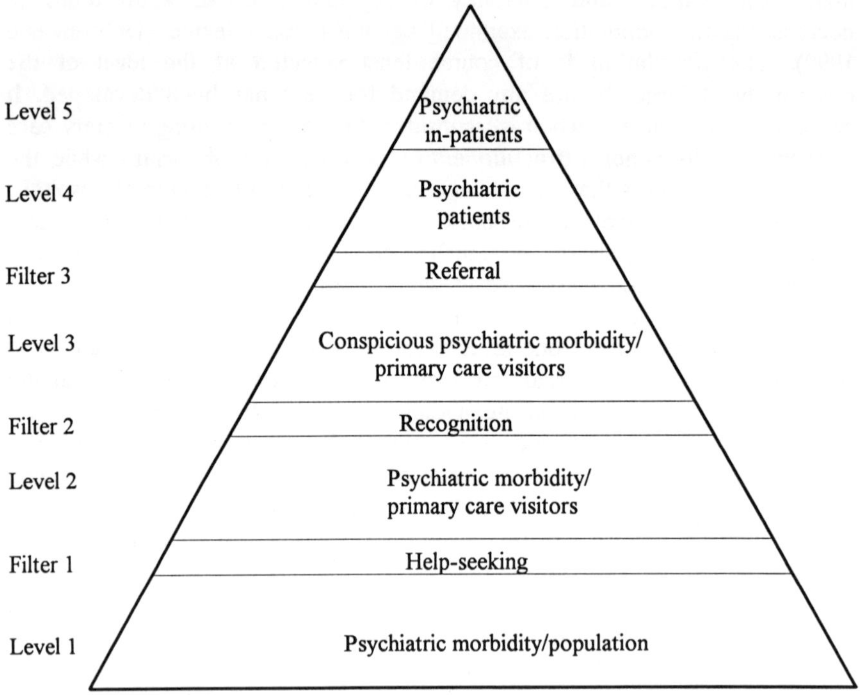

Figure 1.1 Goldberg and Huxley's model

In the above we have already used the term "ideal type". However, a patient will not necessarily always follow this path (c.f. Gater et al. 1991). In health care systems where the general practitioner is not a compulsory intermediary between the patient and the specialist, levels two and three may be omitted. In the Netherlands, a lot of patients apply directly to ambulatory mental health services. There are also but few systems where out-patient psychiatric care services fully control access to the psychiatric hospitals. General Practitioners in the Netherlands regularly decide to admit a patient to a psychiatric hospital, thus eliminating the fourth level.

Nevertheless, broadly speaking the system does work as set out above. This has several notable consequences for the morbidity found at the various levels. In a quantitative sense it means that the higher up the hierarchy we go the smaller the numbers become. After all, the "supply" at each level is dependent on the previous level, and the filters ensure that something "gets left behind" at each level. In a qualitative sense the morbidity undergoes a change at each level. While at the level of the community a relatively high proportion of complaints remain symptoms which do not fit within a nosological syndrome or diagnosis, the more specialized the psychiatric care becomes, the more serious the psychiatric syndromes. Because, apparently, the urge has driven the patient or his environment to pass all these filters. And these serious examples are more outspoken too. See the better performance of diagnostic instruments in clinical settings reported by Dohrenwend. The depressive patients seen by a general practitioner cannot easily be equated with the depressions that are treated in a psychiatric hospital.

The Goldberg and Huxley model as a research model

Goldberg and Huxley's model has been a source of inspiration for a vast amount of psychiatric epidemiological research. By examining epidemiology in such a highly differentiated fashion, Goldberg and Huxley's model has contributed to the fact that the diagnostics employed in general practice and the community are no longer simply extrapolated from those used in psychiatric clinics.

Although their model demands attention for other levels of health care than the traditional psychiatric field, it considers these other levels in the language of the psychiatric disease concept, as we defined this in earlier sections of this chapter. Goldberg and Huxley are searching for psychiatric diagnoses in the community and among general practice visitors, they are comparing diagnoses by general practitioners with the diagnoses made by psychiatrists, etc.

If we are to study the discrepancy between psychiatric epidemiology and the demands put forward by patients, we could consider starting at the level of the population using the patient's frame of reference and ending on the level of the mental hospital using the frame of reference of psychiatry, with the general practitioner's interpretation in between.

In 1972, Bradshaw (cited by de Jong 1986) introduced a useful taxomy to distinguish the several kinds of need, which reflect these different frames of reference. He distinguished:

1) Normative need, need assessed by experts. DSM-III diagnosis are an example of normative need. Results from screening questionnaires being approximations of psychiatric diagnosis are another one. The diagnosis made by the general practitioner should also be regarded as a normative need, the general practitioner being a professional and an

expert too, though at a more general level.

2) Felt need, the need expressed on request by the population, patients, etc. The experience of psychological problems is a felt need.
3) Expressed need/demand, needs which have been translated into a request for help. The complaints put forward by the patient at the doctor's office are regarded as demand.
4) Comparative need, people not receiving help but having the same characteristics as those who do.

As de Jong argues, each approach has its own shortcomings and gives a distorted picture.

Only assessing the normative need results in the inclusion of those people who may share characteristics of clinically disturbed patients but who can cope with it. Consequently they do not translate their sensations in complaints, requiring treatment. Relying solely on the felt need, leads to wrongly attributing a mental illness label to those who are not disturbed enough to justify such a label. On the other hand, people who do not recognize their disturbance as abnormal will be missed. Such is especially the case with patients with a disturbed view of reality.

The same kind of errors are to be expected when the expressed need is taken as point of departure. The false negative error - disturbed patients not seeking help - will even be amplified by factors affecting accessibility.

We can apply this taxonomy to the different perspectives, distinguished by us in the previous pages. When mental disorder is defined in terms of psychiatry we are confronted with normative need. A general practitioner's diagnosis is a normative need as well, but in terms of slightly different rules. The need expressed finally on request by the patient, approaches the mental problems from the viewpoint of the patient. We use the verb "approach" on purpose, because a patient will focus in particular on those experiences which cause a certain amount of concern. When this concern is strong enough, the expressed need might be translated as a demand for help.

Now we may use this terminology to complete the Goldberg and Huxley model.

With such an approach at the first level, the community, the sensation of emotional unwell-being experienced in the population should be measured. We shall label this as the **Felt need**, the need for help experienced by the patient.

At the second and third levels, in other words, general practice, the approach adopted should be based on the patient's request for care. Here **Demand (or expressed need)** is central. The ICPC, in which the Reasons for Encounter are recorded in terms of the patient, is the ideal measuring instrument for this purpose. When this demand is stated in psychosocial terms, the differences between the two levels are not so great, because the patient's explicit request for help with emotional problems is recognized by the general practitioner in almost all cases (Verhaak and Wennink 1990). However, if demand for help is formulated in physical terminology, a difficult process of reattribution is needed, and often discrepancies will remain between patient's experience and the general practitioner's diagnoses. The general practitioner translates the patient's demand into a diagnosis (**Normative need according to the general practitioner**, as set out in either ICPC or ICHPPC). If the diagnosis occasions it, he will refer the patient to a specialist.

The problems that end up at the fourth and fifth levels - generally via the general practitioner - require specialized help. Here the rules of the specialist apply, and he determines what the patient's **Normative need according to the specialist** is, using the terminology of psychiatric syndromes (e.g. DSM-III).

However, the standard method is different in epidemiological research that is based on the filter model. Here, the starting point is the **Normative need according to the specialist** which is the ending point as well. The extent to which this need is present in the general population and in people who consult their general practitioner, and the extent to which it is recognized by general practitioners, as well as what proportion eventually reaches a psychiatrist, are determined in retrospect. Thus it is usual to estimate the incidence of psychiatric problems at the level of the population using GHQ, possibly supplemented by standardized interviews (Goldberg and Huxley 1980, 1992; Giel et al. 1991; Vázquez-Barquero et al. 1990; Williams et al. 1986). In short, the pathway to a psychiatric admission is followed from the viewpoint of the professional and not from that of the demand of the patient.

The crucial point in this matter may be found in the demand for help. Looking for diseases among people who might not be inclined to look for help, might be fruitful in case of diseases which are not recognized in an early stage, which cause serious damage in the long run, and for which an effective therapy exists. Screening for cervical cancer is an example leading him to a diagnosis. In the case of most mental disorders, however, defined by the subjective experience of the patient, it is of little use to consider them as diseases when the patient does not ask for help. In this respect there is a difference between the attitude of a general practitioner and a specialist. It need hardly come as a surprise that a psychiatrist, using a disease model, will try to find symptoms. A general practitioner has a broader view of the patient he knows, with the specific complaint that is troubling him at that moment in time. A general practitioner tries to integrate the demand of the patient within a broader context: "why has this patient come to me now, with this request for help" (c.f. also White 1988). In this respect a general practitioner resembles a psychologist more than a medical specialist such as a psychiatrist. A psychologist, as a specialist with a behavourial background is less interested in underlying diseases but more in patient's style of coping and the relationship between supporting power and burden. Eisenberg (1992) notes that research into general practice should not be directed purely at objective morbidity:

> That service orientation distinguishes research on primary care from epidemiological studies which use symptom counts and cut-off scores to tote up "cases" without reference to disability or to care-seeking behaviour. (Eisenberg 1992, p.4)

This explains why a general practitioner, faced with a patient whose emotional problems he knows, is only inclined to intervene when secondary problems result in the suffering becoming too great.

Although we have objections against solely describing patients on their pathway to psychiatric care in terms of normative needs, the approach of describing each level in its own terminology has the undesirable consequence of incomparability of the several levels. Therefore a combination of terminologies is proposed in the following research questions.

Research questions

This brings us back to the research problem as we defined it at the end of the introductory chapter. We shall have to compare both approaches to learn more about the gap between the observed need according to psychiatric epidemiology and the realized demand for help. And we shall have to use both the concepts of psychiatry as well as those of the lay-man and the general practitioner to arrive at valid conclusions about both the need, met and unmet, at the first three levels of Goldberg and Huxley's model: the population and general practice.

In the introduction we referred to the Dutch National Survey of Morbidity and Interventions in General Practice, which would provide us with the necessary data to undertake such an exercise. In this cross-sectional study we have tried to combine both views by measuring (an approximation of) mental disorder in the "disease - interpretation" and subjective experiences of the same patients as well. These patients will be followed on their "pathway to mental health care", to paraphrase the title of Goldberg and Huxley's work which is already a classic (Goldberg and Huxley 1980). Taking this approach we hope to gain insight into the added value of that part of illness which is not covered by the concept of disease.

In the following research questions we label the mental disorder as a psychiatrist defines it as the "normative need" of a patient. The subjective experience of psychosocial problems is referred to as the "felt need" of the patient. In this book we will look for an answer to the following questions, regarding Doctor's views and Patient's demands:

1. How do felt needs of patients relate to their normative needs as established by psychiatric screening-instruments and with what patient characteristics are felt and normative needs connected?
2. What consequences do felt and normative needs have for help-seeking behaviour[2], and with which characteristics is help-seeking behaviour connected?
3. What demands for help result from felt and normative needs and what characteristics is problem presentation connected with?
4. To what extent are felt and normative needs of patients recognized as such by their general practitioners and how is this related to patient characteristics?
5. How do general practitioners treat the problems of patients with a felt and/or normative need?

When studying this field of tension between felt need and resulting demand for help on the one hand and normative need according to psychiatry on the other hand, patient characteristics influencing the use of medical facilities should be taken into consideration. Andersen and Newman (1973) distinguish three important groups of individual determinants in studying the use of health care facilities:

- predisposing determinants.
- enabling determinants.
- illness level. As illness level (from the point of view of the patient and of the doctor) is already the central concept in our research questions, we shall consider both other kinds of determinants briefly.

In Dutch research on risk-indicators in psychopathology the following characteristics or living conditions are repeatedly mentioned:

- age
- sex
- social economical status
- marital status
- urbanization

Elderly people, women, lower social economical status, singles and people in large cities being more at risk (De Ridder 1988, Ypema and de Haen 1983).

Ormel (1980) concluded that persons out of work because of unemployment or disability run higher risks, together with less well- educated people. Offerhaus (1978), conducting a Dutch study on need for psychiatric help, pointed to the inhabitants of large cities, the widow/widowers, divorced and sick persons as those with the highest risks in this respect.

We conclude from these overviews that we should take the following into consideration as predisposing determinants:

- age
- sex
- marital status
- education
- employment status
- degree of urbanization

Although social economic status is not taken into account directly, it will be highly correlated with level of education and employment status. Almost the same kind of characteristics have been considered in the international literature. (Goldberg and Huxley 1992, Vázquez-Barquero et al. 1990, Williams et al. 1986).

Regarding the enabling determinants: some of the predisposing variables might be considered enabling as well. Education in particular and degree of urbanization might be considered as such, although in different directions. In the case of education, less well-educated people seem to be more at risk of developing mental disorder. Better educated people, on the other hand, being more "protoprofessionalized" (De Swaan 1979) might find it easier to find their way to mental health institutions. In urban areas, mental disorder is more prevalent. On the other hand, in urban areas mental health facilities are more common, thus specialized mental help is more accessible in urban areas. A last enabling determinant to be mentioned is insurance status (private vs public). Publicly insured patients in the Netherlands have fewer financial barriers to primary and specialized health care than (some) privately insured people. We will elaborate on this topic - the Dutch Health Care system- in some detail in the next chapter. However, there is, by definition, a relationship between public insurance and low social economic status, so again the enabling factor outweighs the predisposing one.

In the next chapter we shall consider in detail how the different concepts, summed up in these last pages, have taken shape in our study.

Notes

1. McGuire (1973) gives the following summary of psychiatric research before 1968 when WHO introduced the psychiatric standardization DSM-II.

   Summary of percentage agreement on diagnostic categories between psychiatrists found in several investigations

Authors	No. of pt.	Broad Categories	Specific Categories
Ash (1949)	52	64%	38%
Hunt et al. (1953)	794	54%	32%
Schmidt & Fonda (1956)	426	84%	55%
Kreitman (1961)	90	78%	63%
Beck et al. (1962)	153	70%	54%
Sandifer et al.(1964)	91	73%	57%

   McGuire adds:

   > it may be small consolation to the psychiatrists and psychologists operating within the present classification systems to realise that the position is not significantly different in general medicine. Wilson and Deming (1927) horrified to find only 66 percent agreement on their psychiatric diagnoses, found that this figure was very similar to the agreement between cause of death on the death certificate and the diagnosis arrived at by autopsy. The medical figure was, of course, a validation figure, whereas the psychiatric one was only reliability, in which case the validity is likely to be much less. (p.6)

2. Help-seeking behaviour differs from demand for help in the following way. "Demand" in our research questions implies an explicit demand for help for psychosocial problems. "Help-seeking behaviour" is defined as any contact with professional health care providers, irrespective of the reason for contact. A demand for psychosocial help thus implies help-seeking behaviour, but not the reverse.

2 Methodological background information[1]

Introduction

From April 1987 through March 1988 a large scale study on morbidity and intervention in general practice was conducted in the Netherlands. The study was designed to supply answers to questions concerning the position and function of the Dutch general practitioner. The research was financed by the Ministry of Welfare, Health and Cultural Affairs and the National Council of Sickness Funds.

In a number of respects the survey was inspired by the National Morbidity Surveys held every ten years in England and Wales (Crombie and van der Zee 1982, Royal Coll. Gen. Pract. 1986). They too are aimed at achieving a review of morbidity in general practice, linked with more information about the patients than merely age and sex.

Data from this study serve to provide answers to the questions put forward in the last chapter. In order to interpret these answers correctly it is necessary for the reader to be informed in some detail about the health care system where the data were collected and about the way the study was conducted.

In this chapter both purposes are served. It contains a review of some relevant aspects of the Dutch health care system and a review of the survey design is presented. A review will be given of the data collection methods and the study population covered in this study will be described. Finally the main measuring instruments will be discussed.

The Dutch health care system[2]

General practitioners in the Dutch health care system

The Dutch health care system, as most health care systems in Western Europe is organised on an insurance basis. General practitioners work in a capitation system in the case of publicly insured patients. In contradistinction to many other western European countries, only slightly more than 60% of the Dutch population are insured against costs of medical care on a compulsory basis. This compulsory scheme applies to all employees below a fixed wage level, to old age pensioners who prior to retirement were publicly insured, and to persons in receipt of social benefits. Privately insured persons have a range of insurance options: approximately 70% of privately insured persons have general practitioner coverage.

The payment system for general practitioners differs for publicly and privately insured groups of patients. They receive a fixed sum of money for each publicly insured patient on their lists, irrespective of the number of consultations. Privately insured patients pay the general practitioner directly and are refunded, if covered.

All general practitioners have both privately and publicly insured patients. Publicly insured patients are on the list of general practitioners , while privately insured patients are not, although they usually do consult the same general practitioner.

General practitioners in the Netherlands have a central position as gatekeepers to specialist care, which is only accessible after referral by a general practitioner. Although this is not strictly the case with ambulant mental health care, it is not unusual in these cases too, to require a referral by the general practitioner. Accordingly, most contacts between the public at large and the health care system take place in the general practitioner's practice. The general practitioner decides who is to be referred for further treatment and who is not. Without his permission there are no appointments with medical specialists and without a referral there is no reimbursement of the costs for physical therapy or other paramedical help. Because of this position in the health care system, the general practitioner holds the key to a boundless store of information concerning morbidity patterns as well as the treatment of diseases. For a more elaborate description of the Dutch health care system compared with other systems, see Boerma et al. (1993).

This position of the Dutch general practitioner has the following consequences for patients' pathway to psychiatric care as Goldberg and Huxley outlined it.

Basically there are no financial barriers for most patients to pass the first filter and seek medical help for their problems or complaints. There is a relatively small group (± 10% of the total population) whose primary care costs are not covered. Young, unmarried persons will be overrepresented in this group.

The first filter may be relatively easy to pass, the psychiatrist in a hospital, on the other hand, is mostly not reached without intervention of the general practitioner. In daily practice. especially better educated people, who know where to get therapeutic help, and people with a higher income, who are less dependent on insurance rules, succeed in getting specialist help without a referral. Institutions for ambulatory mental health care (to be discussed below) are more frequently reached without general practitioner intervention.

A last feature of the Dutch health care system which is not without significance for mental health care in primary care is the fixed list. As an average, the Dutch general practitioner sees a patient about four times a year. Each general practitioner keeps a registration system which allows him to combine different medical events and demands for help. What is more, the regular relationship with his patients allows the general practitioner time to test his provisional diagnoses and perhaps time to do its work. As mostly complete families are listed with the same practice, the general practitioner also has the opportunity to get information second-hand and to monitor patients unobtrusively. Of course, all these advantages are much stronger in rural areas with less mobility than urban areas (c.f. Verhey et al. 1992).

Mental health care in the Netherlands

A referral for mental disorder by a general practitioner is in most cases a referral to a more specialized institution for mental health care. We shall discuss the supply and geographical distribution of these facilities below.

Before doing this we have to pay some attention to another opportunity a general practitioner has for such a referral: the social worker. Although a social worker is not considered part of the mental health care system in a restricted sense; since the sixties, the social worker has been an important partner in primary care where treatment of psychosocial problems are concerned. Traditionally social workers applied themselves to marital problems, relational therapy, bereavement groups, in short all kinds of counselling. It appears rather difficult to make a clear distinction between a target group with relatively simple "psychosocial problems" without severe psychopathology to whom social work should be directed and the more severe disorders requiring specialized mental health care (Friele and Verhaak 1991, 1993). Nevertheless, general practitioners do use the social worker as a possible point of referral. Social workers are easy for potential clients to reach, as social work is a community facility with an intricate distribution. In 1993, 166 institutions for social work with 1,227 visiting addresses were reported. They employed 2,914 social workers (staff and executives; Buitink 1993). About twenty-five per cent of all social workers keep regular contact with general practitioners (de Veer 1991). Clients of social work appear to be less well educated and from lower income classes than clients of specialized institutions, to be discussed below (Friele and

Verhaak 1991).

Of the specialized mental health institutions a general practitioner can refer to, the non-residential ones are the most obvious. There are 58 Regional Institutions for Ambulatory Mental Health Care (in Dutch: RIAGG), which are regionally distributed. The catchment area of a RIAGG ranges from 150,000 to 300,000. The professional staff of a RIAGG includes specialized social workers, psychiatrists, social psychiatric nurses and psychologists. In addition, there are psychiatric outpatient clinics, connected to psychiatric hospitals and general hospitals. Of all non-residential mental health care, about 80% was delivered by RIAGGs in 1986 (Bauduin 1988). Although the RIAGGs in more rural areas, in particular, have a decentralized structure with a number of auxiliary branches, out-patient mental health care is in general less easily accessible than primary care in the form of the general practitioner or the social worker. Again, the difference between rural and urban areas - where all services are concentrated - might be of importance in this respect.

The National Study of Morbidity and Interventions

Data collection

The study is based upon three central measuring instruments: the registration of contacts, the patient registration and the patient survey. They will now be discussed in some detail.

Registration of contacts. Over a period of three months the participating general practitioners kept a complete record of the morbidity presented in their practice and of all associated activities.

The contacts registered included face-to-face contacts as well as consultations with receptionists. Consultations by telephone were registered only when they resulted in a repeat prescription or referral.

The registration form included sections on the contacts, on morbidity and also on interventions.

The contact registration form included a number of sections to identify the contact between patient and general practitioner. The following items were recorded:

- point in time when the contact took place (during the day; evening; night)
- length of the consultation;
- nature of the consultation (consultation in the practice; home visits etc);

- initiator of the consultation (patient; general practitioner; someone else);
- type of the consultation (first consultation; repeat consultation; recurrence of disease; periodic check up).

General practitioners were asked to record the reason(s) for the patient's contact and their diagnosis (diagnoses). In one consultation, more than one reason for encounter and diagnosis could occur and, consequently, be recorded. For each diagnosis, the general practitioner recorded the degree to which somatic or psychosocial factors played a role on a 5-point scale.

Reasons for encounter mostly are complaints and symptoms. However, sometimes the reason why the patient visits the doctor is a request for medication or referral while it is also possible that - in a repeat consultation - the patient presents an already established diagnosis as the reason for encounter. The reason for encounter is considered the demand for help.

Reasons for encounter as well as diagnoses recorded by the general practitioner on the registration form had been classified using the International Classification For Primary Care (ICPC) by well trained coders with a medical background. Thus, as regards coding activities the participating general practitioners were not involved themselves, but they were for data quality control.

During the registration period a patient could consult the general practitioner more than once for the same condition. If this happened the diagnoses were linked together into episodes of care. Two possibilities could arise. They were:

- episodes also involving pre-registration period contacts;
- episodes where the first consultation occurred in the registration period; a distinction was made between completely new problems and recurrent problems.

Only the second category of episodes can now be used to calculate incidence statistics; all episode types can be used for calculating the prevalence. Conversion to statistics on a twelve months-basis is possible by quadrupling the incidence rates. Such a solution would result in unreliable statistics for prevalence rates, since chronic conditions exceed the registration period.

As an episode can include several diagnoses, general practitioners have been able to amend the diagnosis in the successive contacts within one episode. For epidemiological purposes it has been decided in general to use the diagnosis of the latest contact to label the episode. Studies on general practitioners interventions, however, are not primarily interested in the final diagnoses but in the diagnosis in every single contact.

The way in which doctors react to the complaints presented, can best be understood from the conclusions on diagnoses drawn at that moment. For that reason the separate diagnosis of every reason for encounter has been stored in the database as well.

General practitioners have recorded the following data on interventions for every reason for encounter:

- requests for laboratory investigations and the results of those investigations;
- activities concerning health promotion, counselling, vaccinations and minor surgery;
- prescriptions for medicines: brand name, strength, daily dose and prescribed dose; prescribed medicines are classified according to the ATC classification;
- referrals to primary and secondary health care providers as well as to hospital; purpose and type (new or repeated) of referral are recorded as well.
- consultations with colleagues and follow up appointments.

Patient registration. It is important to consider the morbidity data against the population at risk and not just against those consulting the general practitioner. Accordingly, information was collected for the whole practice population on the age, sex, marital status, education, sickness insurance type and employment status of the patients registered with the practices of participating general practitioners.

Patient survey and diary. The objectives of the patient survey were to gain information on the morbidity perceived by the population and on factors influencing the presentation of illness to the general practitioner. Indeed, a morbidity registration by general practitioners relates only to reported morbidity, and gives no information on illness not reported to the general practitioner. Moreover, patient registration only provides information on a limited number of patient characteristics.

The survey (a two hour health interview) included several indicators of perceived morbidity: information is collected on recent complaints, on chronic diseases and on psychosocial problems; a disability measure is included as well as the General Health Questionnaire. The survey also includes information on the illness and utilization behaviour of the respondents.

In addition respondents were asked to keep a diary during a period of three weeks in order to furnish insight into the number and kind of health problems for which no professional help was sought.

The current study. In the current study, the several databases were combined. This allows us to consider data from the patient survey and diary together with the registration data from the same patients. In this way we have data at the several levels of the Goldberg & Huxley model, stemming from the same population. As we are only including those above fourteen years of age, this common population counts 10787 persons. For this population we shall present results on mental illness in the community, their help-seeking behaviour, their presentation of psychosocial reasons for visit at the general practitioner's office, their morbidity, as diagnosed by the general practitioner and the treatment of their diseases..

In addition, we shall also present data from the total research population (N=335.000) in the chapters on morbidity and treatment in general practice. In that case, however, we are no longer able to combine these figures with patient characteristics, other than those collected in the patient registration. GHQ and experience of psychological distress reported by the patient can only be combined with morbidity figures of the survey population.

Study population

General practitioners. It was decided to choose a non-proportional stratified sample of general practitioners. A random procedure guaranteed the smallest possible selection. The stratification variables were: degree of urbanization, region and distance from the hospital. Four degrees of urbanization were distinguished according to the classification of the Dutch Central Statistical Bureau; three regions (the northern, the middle and the southern part of the country) and three distance groups (the doctor's surgery is in the immediate vicinity of a hospital, his surgery is at a distance of between 0 and 15 km from a hospital, or the distance to the nearest hospital is over 15 km). Non-proportional stratification guaranteed that all values of the stratification variables were well represented in the sample. The sample was drawn from the NIVEL file of general practitioners practising as principals on 01-01-1985.

General practitioners were invited to participate in the study by means of a letter accompanied by a recruitment folder and letters of recommendation from the Dutch GPs Association and the National College of general practitioners. It must be emphasized that general practitioners themselves were approached, and not the practices as such.

Colleagues of general practitioners in the sample working in the same surgery, were also requested to participate for several reasons. In the first place the age-sex register was linked to the practice as a whole and often not to the doctors as individuals. Furthermore, patients often visit more than one general practitioner in a practice. As it was our aim to link reasons for encounter to episodes of care, the morbidity presented to these colleagues was indispensable.

In a limited number of the stratification cells it was necessary to accept the participation of general practitioner volunteers.

161 general practitioners participated in the study. The average age of the doctors taking part in the study was lower than the national average; more female general practitioners participated, and fewer doctors working in single handed practices. These general practitioners were paid for their participation.

Patients. On the patient side some basic information was gathered on the total patient population of the participating general practitioners. In addition, supplementary information was collected in a random sample of 100 patients per participating general practitioner by means of a health interview study (the patient survey).

For each practice an age/sex patient register was set up. The study covered a population of approx. 335 000 patients treated by the participating general practitioners. There was a high level of correspondence on both age and sex distributions.

Background and social data was collected by means of the patient registration for the total patient group. It was possible to collect information for about 90% of the total patient group. Nevertheless, this response percentage differed depending upon the questions asked. Non response was higher for indicators of social class such as education and occupation. In addition to this patient registration, a random sample of 100 patients on the list of every general practitioner participating in the study was invited to take part in a health interview study and a health diary covering a three week period. Thus, patients selected for the interview did not necessarily have to have visited their general practitioner to be selected for the interview. Patients of all ages were selected. The response rate for the health interview was 76%, including 13,014 completed interviews. Nearly 93% of the respondents participating in this interview also completed the health diary. The age/sex distribution of the patients participating in the health interview study shows only small differences with the total Dutch population: the number of respondents in the 25-44 age group is slightly overrepresented.

Operationalization of crucial concepts

In the last chapter, we have introduced the concepts "felt need", "normative need", and "general practitioner's diagnosis". The operationalization of these concepts and the ideas behind it deserve some clarification.

Felt need Felt need comprises the problems and problem situations as the patient experiences them. Felt need exists irrespective of whether (medical) help has been sought for or not. It is the condition of the patient in the so-called pre-medical stage. As we know from population studies, only about ten per cent of all physical and psychological complaint leads to a request for professional help (vd Lisdonk 1988).

Felt need might be measured by open questions (for example Furer en Tax 1987) but results from such an approach may be hard to compare. Consequently, a list of 65 acute physical and psychological complaints and problems was handed out to the respondents during the health interview, requiring them to indicate the complaints and problems experienced during the past two weeks. Eight items indicated a psychological or social complaint/problem; if one or more of those were indicated, the respondent was considered to have experienced a "felt psychosocial need".

A disadvantage of such a measurement is that it invites people to complain. This invitation to complain is more or less inherent to the interview method. Fortunately, all participants to the health interview were also requested to keep a health diary during three weeks. All physical and psychosocial complaints, experienced during this period, were to be registered by the respondent in this diary. This was to be in the respondent's own words, which were classified afterwards. Each respondent noting at least one problem or complaint classified as "psychological" or "social" was regarded as having experienced a "felt psychosocial need". In this way the subjective experience of being unwell is reported strictly at the patient's initiative.

A last indicator was the recent experience of psychosocial stressful events. It was measured by the Biographical Problem Inventory (Biopro), originally developed by Mooney as the Mooney Problem List (1950), later adapted by Furer and Tax (1987). It contains 22 items, about relational, social and psychological problem situations which are recently experienced. If a respondent had experienced one or more problematic situations, his score on the Biopro was considered positive. It should be mentioned that the Biopro is not so much an indicator of need, as one of the psychological burdens a patient is experiencing and as such a possible predictor for "felt psychosocial need".

Demand The demand for help as it is expressed by the patient, was registered by the general practitioner during each contact and coded afterwards in the ICPC. Patients reporting at least one complaint within ICPC-chapter "Psychological" or "Social" were considered to be expressing a psychosocial demand for help.

Normative need We defined "the mental disorder as a professional defines it as normative need". As we saw in the foregoing chapter, nowadays the most sophisticated way of assessing a person's psychiatric status is by a standardized psychiatric interview. Such an approach has been followed in the American Epidemiological Catchment Area studies, but is in general too expensive. Because of this drawback, the two stage sampling approach has been developed, in which case a screening instrument precedes the standardized interview, to be held with only a small sub-sample of the original sample. The interview serves the function of calibrating the screening test.

In many cases the GHQ is used as screening test, and as a result the GHQ is very well documented, regarding its sensitivity and specificity. Goldberg (1985) reports figures for specificity ranging from .73 - .93 and for sensitivity from .67 - 1. The positive predictive value ranges from .55 to .75.[3]

An objection against such screening-lists in general and the GHQ in particular is its possible contamination with general feelings of demoralization and physical unwell-being. As Dohrenwend et al. (1980) pointed it, "elevated scores on these scales tell you that something is wrong". It does not necessarily mean that that "something" is associated with psychopathology and on the other hand, some psychopathology may be possible without non-specific psychological distress the screening lists are measuring. DeMarco (1984), reporting on the physiological and psychological dimensions on the Langner-22 item scale (a comparable screening test), concludes that his results

> strongly support the interpretation that the scale measures primarily one major dimension which ... can be presumed to be mild undifferentiated psychopathology (DeMarco 1984, p.64).

This conclusion is based on the results that both physical and psychological symptoms of the scale made an effective contribution in differentiating subjects at risk from controls, that all the items correlated substantially with the total score and therefore are likely to measure the same underlying trait, and that Cronbach's alpha of .86 indicated the existence of one dimension. Nevertheless, in case of this Langner scale, caution was required because of low specificities. Ormel et al., (1989) analyzing longitudinal data in which both GHQ-28 and PSE-score were available, conclude that the GHQ indicated the changes in severity, the PSE was measuring.

These considerations, combined with the fact that the GHQ is often used in the international literature as an indicator for psychopathology, make it legitimate to use the GHQ, as assessed during the health interview, as an indicator for the "normative need" of the patient. Because, it seems plausible to assume that an important part of the respondents, scoring high on the GHQ, would have been diagnosed as mentally disturbed by a psychiatrist, had he been interviewing the respondent concerned. We should be aware however of the possible contamination with physical unwell-being.

Another point of consideration is the assessment of the GHQ on one particular point in time, while following the respondents during a three month period. This issue will be considered if necessary.

GP's diagnosis The "normative need" from the point of view of the general practitioner has been registered by the general practitioner on the occasions that patients visited his office during the registration period. The general practitioner gave a diagnosis which was coded in the ICPC. Furthermore, the general practitioner assessed each diagnosis on a 5-point scale, ranging from "completely somatic" to "completely psychological". This provided the general practitioner with the occasion to evaluate diagnoses which fell into categories like "gastro-intestinal" or "neurological" also with an evaluation that the abdominal pain or headache was not entirely a physical matter in his eyes.

Figure 2.1 summarizes the indicators for need and demand and the samples in which they have been measured.

	Population > 14 year 268.000 enlisted patients	Interview > 14 year Sample of 10.787 enlisted patients
Felt need		Acute psychological complaints reported in interview Psychological complaints reported in diary Recent stressful life events
Demand	Reason for Encounter, stated by the patient, coded in ICPC	
Normative need (psychiatrist)		Score on the GHQ, assessed during interview
Normative need (GP)	- Diagnosis coded in the ICPC - 5-point scale (completely somatic - completely psychological) assessment of each diagnosis	
Background characteristics	Age, Sex, Educational level, Marital status, Employment status, Insurance, Urbanization	

Note: As the interview sample is a sub-sample from the population, all variables available in population sample are also available in interview sample, but not the other way around.

Figure 2.1 Core variables in the study as measured in population and in interview samples respectively

Notes

1. The information of this chapter is derived from Foets, M., Velden J. van der, Bakker D. de, Dutch National Survey of General Practice - A Summary of the Survey Design. Utrecht, NIVEL, 1992.

2. The situation as it existed during the data gathering of the National Study ('87-'88) will be described.

3. Specificity can be defined as the proportion of "true non-cases" not correctly identified by the screening test. Sensitivity is the proportion of "true cases" which is correctly identified as a case by the test. Predictive value is the proportion "true cases" among those identified by the test as a case. The relationship between a test's score (T) and the probable "real" prevalence (P) is dependent on the test's sensitivity and specificity and can be expressed in the following equation (Goldberg and Huxley, 1980):

   $$P = (T - (1\text{-specificity}))/(\text{sensitivity} - (1\text{-specificity}))$$

   When we assume the average specificity for the GHQ to be .80 and the average sensitivity .85, the equation goes:

   $$P = (T - .20)/(.85 - .20) \text{ or } P = 1.54T - .31$$

   It can be concluded that a GHQ's test score with such test-characteristics is only a raw approximation (and usually an overestimation) of the true prevalence. This is mainly due to the relatively large proportion of people who are indicated wrongly by the GHQ as probable cases of mental disorder.

3 Mental disorder in the population and help-seeking behaviour

Introduction

Subject of this chapter are felt need and normative need in the population, or, in other words, mental disorder as it is experienced by the persons in question and as it is assessed by psychiatric screening methods. Furthermore, the resulting help-seeking behaviour will be considered. First, evidence from the literature on this topic will be discussed. Next, results from our own survey will be presented.

A review of literature on mental disorder in the population

The psychiatric perspective: normative need in the population

As has been illustrated in chapter 1, recent psychiatric epidemiological research in the population (i.e. among people who have not already been selected by seeking help) is generally carried out by means of a two-stage sampling approach. Among large representative samples a first screening instrument (such as the General Health Questionnaire (GHQ) or Symptom Check List (SCL-90) is administered. In the second shift, proportioned subsamples are questioned, using standardized psychiatric interviews, like the Present State Examination (PSE) or the Diagnostic Interview Schedule (DIS). Many psychiatric morbidity statistics are based on GHQ, DIS or PSE. In this review we shall consider recent findings of these kind of surveys.

GHQ-research Figure 3.1 (next page) summarizes prevalence rates as they are measured by the GHQ. In most surveys where the probability of mental disturbance was estimated using this screening-instrument prevalence rates between 150 and 250 per 1000 population were reported. Women are generally more at risk than men, and divorce or unemployment enlarges the chances considerably. The several studies are inconclusive about age-effects: Finlay-Jones and Burvill (1977) and Williams et al. (1986) report more young people (up to forty years of age) as potential cases than older people, while Vázquez-Barquéro et al. (1990) find an increase with age.

Investigator	Prev/1000	♂ : ♀	Details
Finlay-Jones and Burvill (1977) GHQ-60 Australia	163	1:1.4	N = 2324 Peak ♂, age 30-39; ♀, age 15-29. Divorced > married, widowed or single people. ♂ lower SES > ♂ higher SES
Goldberg, Kay Thompson (1974) GHQ-60 UK	184	1:2	N = 213
Hodiamont et al. (1987) GHQ-30 The Netherlands	227	1:1.1	N = 3232
v. Limbeek et al. (1994) The Netherlands	254		N = 2628 Large city population > 18 year
Vázquez-Barquero et al. (1990) GHQ-60 Spain	185	1:2.1	N = 1223 increase with age. High for divorced and unemployed ♂
Williams et al. 1986 GHQ-30 UK	234	1:1.2	N = 3314 High risk for young ♂ (<30yr.). Also for unemployed ♂, divorced ♀ and middle class ♀.

Figure 3.1 Prevalence rates per 1000 population at risk for random samples of the general population; based on direct assessment by the GHQ

Moreover, Vázquez-Barquéro et al. (1990) and Williams et al. (1986) reported more general practitioner contacts by people scoring above GHQ-threshold, compared with those scoring below threshold.

Population surveys with PSE The PSE is usually administered in relatively small samples together with the GHQ. By means of logistical regression, models are fitted to estimate from the GHQ-score the prevalences of PSE-diagnoses in the larger population. As the sensitivity and specificity of the

GHQ in relationship with the PSE is not perfect, prevalences measured by the PSE tend to be lower than GHQ prevalences.

Hodiamont et al. (1987) followed this procedure and found 72/1000 male PSE-cases and 75/1000 female cases in a Dutch survey. These results were compared by them with Australian data (Henderson 1979), where 90/1000 cases were found for both sexes. The probability of being a PSE-case were higher for elderly people, the divorced and widows/widowers, the less well-educated, the unemployed and the chronically ill.

Lethinen et al. (1990), doing the same in Finland, found 174/1000 PSE-cases (145/1000 male, 196/1000 female), a prevalence increasing with age.

Vázquez-Barquéro et al. (1987, 1988) report a total prevalence of 147/1000 PSE-cases, being 81/1000 male and 206/1000 female.

Population research with DIS: the Epidemiological Catchment Area (ECA) Surveys The ECA-surveys are large-scale psychiatric epidemiological investigations in five locations in the United States of America (Robins and Regier 1990). These results deserve special attention because for all respondents (19.640) a complete DIS-interview could be assessed. The DIS, as the PSE, can be regarded as a real diagnostic instrument, in contradistinction to the GHQ which only provides an estimate of the probability of mental disorder. The PSE results, mentioned above, were based on estimates of the GHQ. The DIS, however, was administered to all respondents, involved in the ECA study.

Myers et al. (1984) reported preliminarily 72/1000 to 86/1000 respondents with a DSM-III diagnosis during the two weeks before the interview. These rates increase when a longer time-span has been taken into consideration, cumulating in a lifelong prevalence of 230/1000 to 252/1000[1].

The definite report (Robins and Regier 1990) concluded at 200/1000 people with an active disorder last year and with 320/1000 people having experienced a mental disorder once in their lives. In a later refinement, on the basis of a follow-up one year later, Regier et al. (1993) corrected the one-year prevalence in 280/1000 (220/1000 without addiction). The odds are higher for women, for younger people, the separated and divorced and the socially deprived.

ECA-data have been used to study help-seeking behaviour of mentally disturbed people. Persons with a DSM-III diagnosis visit medical doctors more frequently than persons without a diagnosis. Leaf and Bruce (1987) and Shapiro et al. (1984) reported more women seeking help in case of a diagnosis than men. Women tended to seek help from non-specialized agencies, such as family doctors. Men, on the other hand, were more likely to go to specialized mental health services, to see psychiatrists and mental health centres. Older patients only rarely visited a specialized agency.

The patient's perspective: felt need

Mooney's Problem Inventory has been used in Dutch research to inventarize the problem situations experienced. It is a measure for the mental burden, not necessarily concomitant with mental distress, but very often related to it[2]. The inventory measures the prevalence of problems in 22 different domains (work, finance, relationship, education, addiction etc.).

In the Dutch Nijmegen Regional Study (Furer and Tax 1987), 25% did not experience any problem situations, 35% experienced problems in one or two domains and 40% in three domains or more.

In other research, patients were asked directly about their feelings of mental distress, without any standardization. Lehtinen et al. (1990) asked the respondents in their population survey if they considered psychiatric treatment necessary, a question which was answered affirmatively (absolutely or probably) by 7.3%. 1.5% felt sure that they needed psychiatric help. More women than men felt themselves in need of treatment and this feeling was highest in the 50 to 60 age group. This self-assessed need could be compared with PSE estimations. 28% of those who were diagnosed as "psychotic", 11% of those with a diagnosis of "depression" and only 5% of those respondents with an other diagnosis felt themselves in absolute need of treatment.

In the Nijmegen Regional Study patients reported on negative feelings during the preceding week by completing the Affective Balance Scale, developed by Bradburn (1969) The ABS has five positive and five negative items, the negative ones asking if "you have been very lonesome / restless / bored / depressed / agitated during the past weeks". One third of the respondents had not experienced any negative feeling, five per cent responded affirmatively to all five questions.

Conclusions from the literature

Point prevalence of psychiatric disturbance, measured by screening instruments is between 15% and 25% of the population. Structured psychiatric diagnostic interviews result in point prevalences of about 10%. Prevalence rates increase substantially when longer periods are considered.
All these rates reflect the viewpoint of the psychiatrist.

From the point of view of the patient we can conclude that many people experience feelings of disturbance or problem situations, but only a few consider themselves in need of psychiatric treatment, even when a psychiatric diagnosis has been established. In this respect the results of Hodiamont et al. (1986) discussed in chapter 1 are relevant: most patients with a psychiatric diagnosis experience negative feelings, but only a small number of those who have experienced negative feelings received a psychiatric diagnosis.

As was mentioned in the previous chapters, mental disorder within our research population has been assessed from each of the perspectives, discussed here. In the next part of this chapter we will express the prevalence of mental disturbance in the study population in the following ways:

- by measurement of feelings of mental disturbance, experienced during the previous two weeks
- diary notes during the previous three weeks
- by measurement of number of psychosocial domains in which problem situations exist
- by using the GHQ-score, as an approximation of the result of a psychiatric examination.

Mental problems in the population: prevalence and patient characteristics

Felt need in the population: the experience of psychosocial complaints and feelings of mental distress

Positive responses on check-list. People experience a lot of complaints and problems in the short time span of fourteen days. Table 3.1 gives the proportion of respondents that indicated each item, when questioned about it during the interview. The psychosocial items are presented first in line[3].

When we take the eight psychosocial problems together, 4051 respondents (37.6% of the population) indicated they had experienced one or more of these complaints. About half of them had experienced one psychosocial problem, one quarter had experienced two of the psychosocial complaints mentioned, fourteen per cent had experienced three complaints and fourteen per cent had experienced four or more complaints. In the following analyses we distinguish between respondents who did not report any psychosocial complaints and respondents who reported at least one.

Table 3.1
Experienced complaints in a 2-week period (N=10787)

Psychosocial complaints:			
Nervous	20%	Sleeplessness	16%
Easily agitated	15%	Listlessness	12%
Aggressive feelings	7%	Problems at work	3%
Family problems	3%	Chronically nervous	0%
Physical complaints:			
Headache	32%	Tiredness	31%
Stuffy nose	20%	Cough	20%
Complaints back	19%	Complaints neck/shoulder	16%
Complaints leg/knee/foot	14%	Sore throat	12%
Dizziness	11%	Excessive perspiration	11%
Complaints hand/finger	11%	Hearing difficulty	10%
Tightness of the chest	8%	Oppressed in chest	8%
Abdominal cramp	8%	Compl. Bowel movement	7%
Ringing in the ear	7%	Heartburn	7%
Stomachache	6%	Complaints hip	6%
Heart palpitations	6%	Nausea	6%
Increase in weight	6%	Swollen ankles	5%
Diarrhoea	5%	Menstrual pain	5%
Fever	4%	Earache	4%
Toothache	4%	Vomiting	3%
Incontinence	3%	Nose bleeding	2%
Eating problem	2%	Burning feeling on urination	2%

Table 3.2 gives the distribution of characteristics. Experience of psychosocial complaints increases with age, among women as well as among men. Female respondents in general experience more psychosocial complaints than men.

Widows/widowers and divorced respondents, people who have suffered a loss, report far more psychosocial complaints than married persons or those who have never been married.

Although there are differences between the various educational levels, this relationship is not a linear one. One could say that those who had technical or vocational training as their highest level of education reported fewer psychosocial complaints than those with only primary school and those with a secondary or tertiary.

Employment status has a clear effect on the experience of feelings of mental disturbance. Those who are still studying and those who have paid employment have the least psychosocial complaints. Those who run a household or who no longer have a employment report psychosocial complaints much more frequently. Those who are out of work because of disability experience psychosocial complaints very frequently.

Table 3.2
Proportion of respondents who experienced psychosocial complaints, with different background characteristics

		Men		Women	
		N	%	N	%
Sex		5284	31%	5503	44% •
Age	15-24	1031	26.1%	1077	39.4% •
	25-44	2263	29.3%	2275	39.4%
	45-64	1387	35.3%	1346	50.1%
	65-74	429	29.8%	514	53.5%
	75+	174	43.1%	291	53.6%
				N	%
Marital status	Married			6793	35.7% •
	Divorced			395	59.5%
	Widows/widowers			630	54.9%
	Unmarried			2969	35.2%
Highest level of education completed	Primary school only			3030	42.8% •
	Techn./Voc Training 12-16 yrs			2739	34.6%
	Lower general second. education			1467	37.0%
	Techn./Voc Training 16-18 yrs			1307	32.0%
	Higher general second. education			654	37.9%
	Techn./Voc Training 18+			867	36.4%
	University			212	36.8%
Employment status	Student/Conscript			2489	34.5% •
	Housewife/man			1482	43.3%
	Unemployed			232	43.5%
	Incapacitated			334	60.2%
	Retired			1348	44.5%
	Working			3826	32.5%
Insurance	Public			7237	39.4% •
	Private			3475	33.8%
Urbanization	Rural			4196	34.2% •
	Suburban			4320	36.5%
	Urban			1673	44.1%
	3 Large cities			549	49.9%

• $p < .0001$ (chi-square)

Insurance also has an effect: those who are publicly-insured have a higher rate of psychosocial complaints than privately-insured respondents.

Finally, people experience more psychosocial distress, when they live in a more urbanized environment. About one third of those living in the countryside report psychosocial complaints, while almost half of all the inhabitants of the three large cities in the Netherlands (Amsterdam, Rotterdam, The Hague) do so.

Of course, there are a number of interrelationships between these characteristics: widows/widowers and divorced people are older in general than married people and those who are as yet unmarried. The age-sex distribution for employment status certainly is not equal, privately-insured people are older, but have also a higher level of education and a better employment status. To get a better insight in these interactions, a multivariate analysis has been carried out. In such an analysis the effects of each parameter is estimated, while controlling for the effect of the others. The logistic regression is given at the end of the chapter[4].

After controlling for others variables, the effect of the education-level disappeared. Among the categories of marital status, being a widow/widowers does not exercise any effect. Being divorced, on the other hand, considerably increases the probability of experiencing psychosocial complaints. Among the several categories of employment status unemployment and being incapacitated are the important factors.

When we consider all the determinants together, we might state that people in general experience psychosocial complaints when they are older, female, divorced, publicly-insured, living in an urbanized area and/or out of work (be it because of disability or not). In the case of disabled people (compared to working people), the divorced (compared to unmarried people), women (compared to men) and people from large cities (compared to those living in rural areas) the chances are considerably higher (more than 1.7 times as much).

Psychological complaints in the diary. Although about one third of the respondents indicated experience of psychosocial complaints, only fifteen per cent of those who kept a diary during three weeks after the interview recorded psychological complaints during one or more of these days. Most of them are coded as "stress".

Although there is a certain overlap between those who answered the question as to whether they had experienced certain psychological problems affirmatively and those who spontaneously recorded those problems in a diary, only thirty per cent of the former belonged to the latter and sixty per cent of the latter to the former. We cannot speak of the "problem-recorders" as being a selection of the larger group who complain on request.

The characteristics of those who recorded psychological complaints in their diary, given in table 3.3 are also slightly different from the characteristics of those who reported psychosocial complaints.

Again, women more frequently record psychological problems than men. The effect of urbanization is also comparable in its effect on the experience of psychosocial problems, reported during the interview. With respect to employment status, maintaining a household means a risk in respect of paid employment, but being disabled leads to a comparable probability and those who are unemployed or retired run less risk of psychological complaints in their diary than the working people. Divorced people in both cases (interview and diary) run a higher risk of mental problems, but widows and widowers do not distinguish themselves in their diary to the extent they did when questioned about their mental problems.

When people are asked to record their psychological complaints spontaneously, overrepresentation of the 25-44 age group, the better educated and the privately-insured is found. This is contrary to the findings from the interview, where psychological problems increased with age, decreased with education and were more abundant for publicly-insured.

Taking all the effects together, women, the better-educated, the disabled, divorced and the inhabitants of urban areas are significantly more likely to record mental problems in their diary. The regression table is given in the notes at the end of the chapter[5]. From the high odds ratios for the better educated, as well as from the disappearance of effects of greater age, unemployment and public insurance we might cautiously conclude that the method of measurement has somehow been of influence on the results.

Table 3.3
Proportion of respondents who recorded psychosocial complaints, in their diary with different background characteristics

		Men N	Men %	Women N	Women %
Sex		4879	12.5%	5034	22.8% *
Age	15-24	970	10.6%	1028	21.1% *
	25-44	2112	14.1%	2148	25.5%
	45-64	1287	12.7%	1225	21.9%
	65-74	384	9.1%	437	18.1%
	75+	126	6.3%	196	17.9%

		N	%
Marital status	Married	6327	16.8% *
	Divorced	339	28.9%
	Widows/widowers	487	18.7%
	Unmarried	2760	18.1%
Highest level of completed education	Primary school only	2689	13.5% *
	Techn./Voc Training 12-16 yrs	2585	14.3%
	Lower general second. education	1373	20.3%
	Techn./Voc Training 16-18 yrs	1232	20.2%
	Higher general second. education	596	23.8%
	Techn./Voc Training 18+	800	28.0%
	University	189	31.7%
Employment status	Student/Conscript	2254	15.5% *
	Housewife/man	1399	22.2%
	Unemployed	213	14.1%
	Incapacitated	303	19.1%
	Retired	1142	14.1%
	Working	3621	18.6%
Insurance	Public	6625	17.0% **
	Private	3220	19.0%
Urbanization	Rural	3925	15.4% *
	Suburban	3997	16.8%
	Urban	1530	22.7%
	3 Large cities	461	27.8%

* $p < .0001$ ** $p < .05$ (chi-square)

Keeping a health diary might have been easier for those who are more used to expressing themselves through the spoken and the written word.

Presence of potential problem situations in the population

52% of the respondents indicated at least one psychosocial domain which could be characterized as being troublesome. The most frequently indicated domains were "bad prospects for the future", "changes in society", "one"s self image" and "impossibility for self-development". Each of these situations was indicated by 12 to 16% of the respondents. Material problem situations ("work", "financing", "housing", "living situation") were each indicated by 6 to 8% Relationships ("parents", "partner", "children" , "other relationships") were problematic in one way or another for 13%.

Table 3.4 shows the existence of problem situations for respondents with different characteristics. More women than men had at least one problem situation. Differences between age-groups are not that large, although statistically significant. For both sexes the 65-74 age group catches the eye by having the least persons with problem situations.

The divorced and widows/widowers notably often experience problem situations, as do the unemployed and incapacitated respondents.

People in the city not only experience more psychosocial complaints, they also report more troublesome situations than people from rural and suburban areas.

Finally, the effect of education is striking, because the number of persons with problems increase with level of education. Problems in personal relations contribute significantly to this tendency.

Taking all the effects together in a multivariate analysis, the risk of problem situations is significantly higher for the divorced and widows/widowers, for women, for the better educated, those living in urbanized areas and for the unemployed or disabled. The risk is significantly lower for retired people. The regression table is given in the notes at the end of the chapter[6]

Table 3.4
Proportion of respondents with at least one problem situation

		Men		Women	
		N	%	N	%
Sex		5186	49.6%	5396	54.9% •
Age	15-24	1005	46.0%	1052	53.1% •
	25-44	2232	51.2%	2237	56.8%
	45-64	1364	51.5%	1321	55.0%
	65-74	417	41.0%	501	50.9%
	75+	168	54.2%	285	53.3%
				N	%
Marital status	Married			6793	35.7% •
	Divorced			395	59.5%
	Widows/widowers			630	54.9%
	Unmarried			2969	35.2%
Highest level of completed education	Only primary school			2965	50.9% •
	Techn./Voc Training 12-16 yrs			2690	48.8%
	Lower general second. education			1438	51.7%
	Techn./Voc Training 16-18 yrs			1289	54.1%
	Higher general second. education			643	58.8%
	Techn./Voc Training 18+			858	57.2%
	University			208	66.8%
Employment status	Student/Conscript			2427	50.3% •
	Housewife/man			1459	55.6%
	Unemployed			229	71.6%
	Incapacitated			323	62.8%
	Retired			1318	47.9%
	Working			3764	51.1%
Insurance	Public				
	Private				
Urbanization	Rural			4132	48.2% •
	Suburban			4226	52.5%
	Urban			1641	58.3%
	3 Large cities			534	65.2%

• $p < .0001$ (chi-square)

Figure 3.2 presents the distribution of the scores on the GHQ among the respondents. We use the cut-off point of 4/5, as is common with the 30-item version of the GHQ. 9.3% of the male respondents and 15.7% of the women score above threshold and are to be considered potential cases of mental disturbance. Distribution of other characteristics are given in table 3.5

The GHQ increases with age for male respondents, except for the 65-74 age group, where the line is interrupted. For females the relationship is curvilinear with a peak for the 45-64 years age group.

Thc divorced and widows/widowers clearly have an increased probability of psychopathology, according to the GHQ.

There is no clear relationship between educational level and proportion of GHQ-caseness. On the other hand, the probability of a score above the threshold for certain categories of the unemployed (in the first place the disabled, but also unemployed and housewives) is markedly higher than for people with paid employment. Publicly-insured people have a higher risk on a high GHQ-score than the privately-insured. People from urbanized areas have a higher average GHQ-score than people from rural and suburban arcas.

After logistic regression, four of them remain keeping an independent effect. These are: marital status, sex, urbanization and employment status[7].

Other variables remained constant, women, divorced and widows/widowers persons, people from large cities and people who are out of work are at a greater risk of being considered a potential case of mental illness.

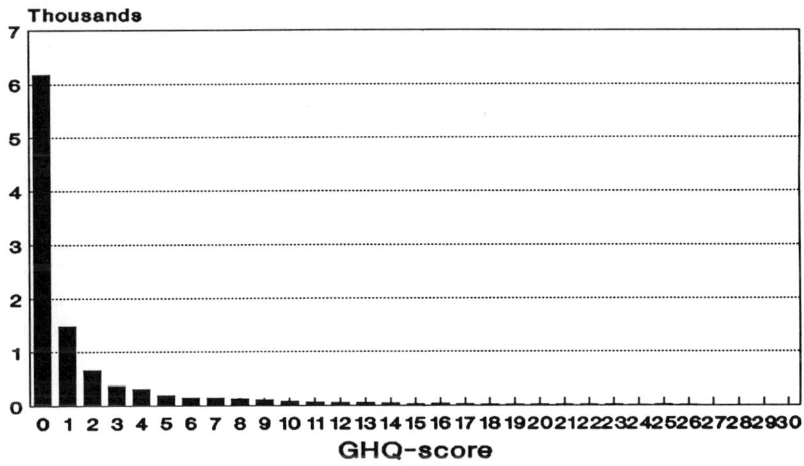

Figure 3.2 Distribution of GHQ-scores

Table 3.5
Proportion of respondents, scoring above GHQ-threshold, according to their characteristics

		Men N	Men %	Women N	Women %
Sex		5092	9.3%	5213	15.7% *
Age	15-24	990	6.8%	1015	14.8%***
	25-44	2184	9.6%	2158	16.0%
	45-64	1340	10.8%	1265	16.4%
	65-74	414	6.8%	498	15.7%
	75+	164	13.4%	277	14.4%

		N	%
Marital status	Married	6469	11.5% *
	Divorced	370	25.6%
	Widows/widowers	606	18.2%
	Unmarried	2833	12.0%
Highest level of completed education	Primary school only	2894	14.0%***
	Techn./Voc Training 12-16 yrs	2616	11.9%
	Lower general second. education	1407	11.8%
	Techn./Voc Training 16-18 yrs	1230	10.6%
	Higher general second. education	628	14.0%
	Techn./Voc Training 18+	844	12.1%
	University	209	12.4%
Employment status	Student/Conscript	2364	11.5% *
	Housewife/man	1404	16.1%
	Unemployed	227	18.5%
	Incapacitated	317	24.0%
	Retired	1296	12.3%
	Working	3671	10.4%
Insurance	Public	7237	13.4% **
	Private	3475	10.8%
Urbanization	Rural	4040	10.7%
	Suburban	4080	12.7%
	Urban	1618	14.7%
	3 Large cities	519	18.9%

* $p < .0001$ ** $p < .001$ *** $p < .05$ (chi-square)

Felt need, problem situations and normative need compared

There is a certain kind of overlap between the three indicators derived from the health interview, as is illustrated in Figure 3.3.

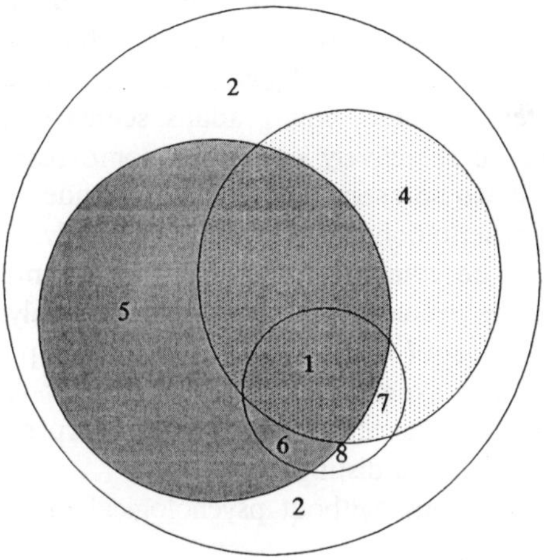

9.7%	1:	GHQ + SYMP + BIOPRO +
36.5%	2:	GHQ - SYMP - BIOPRO -
24%	3:	GHQ - SYMP - BIOPRO +
9.8%	4:	GHQ - SYMP + BIOPRO -
17.1%	5:	GHQ - SYMP + BIOPRO +
1.5%	6:	GHQ + SYMP - BIOPRO +
1.0%	7:	GHQ + SYMP + BIOPRO -
.4%	8:	GHQ + SYMP - BIOPRO -

Figure 3.3 Overlap between problem situations, experienced psycho-social complaints and GHQ

These three indicators all reflect the response to an invitation to express precoded complaints. Figure 3.3 shows a hierarchy between these three indicators. Many people experience problem situations, quite a lot of them have had feelings of mental distress, and a relative minority scores above threshold on the GHQ. Problematic situations appear to be a necessary - but not a sufficient - prerequisite for feelings of mental distress, which in turn were a necessary, but again not sufficient condition for a high GHQ-score. In other words: not all need, expressed on request, will be assessed as a need by experts.

More than one third did not refer to any problem situation, did not experience psychological distress and scored below threshold on the GHQ. Another quarter mentioned problem situations without referring to psychological distress or scoring high on the GHQ. Seventeen per cent combined problem situations with psychological distress, without being a GHQ-case. Ten per cent of the population are positive on all three indicators. Thus, this hierarchy holds true for 87.3% of all respondents. The majority of those who do not comply with this hierarchy are people who report psychological distress without indicating any problematic situation. Of all GHQ-cases, 85% also reported psychological distress and 89% indicated at least one problem situation.

However, the records in the diary do not fit within this hierarchy. Too many people, more than thirty per cent, recording emotional problems in their diary, did not express psychological distress during the interview. The same holds true for the GHQ-diary relationship. The diary data are of another order: they are spontaneously expressed and therefore, a better reflection of the patient's need of feeling of subjection. On the other hand, the overrepresentation of better educated, young adults seems to indicate that such an expression might be selectively easier for some respondents than for others. In each case, it would seem advisable to consider the help seeking behaviour and illness presentation of this group separately.

The other three indicators can be combined. This has the advantage that the different groups are mutually exclusive. In the foregoing analyses one had to take in mind that the group of GHQ-positive persons is partly the same as the group of persons who experienced psychosocial problems. By making mutual exclusive groups differences can be better interpreted. The following four groups of respondents are distinguished:

1) People without problem situations, without psychological distress, and GHQ below five.
2) People who have experienced at least one problem situation, without psychological distress, and GHQ below five.
3) People who have experienced at least one problem situation, with psychological distress, and GHQ below five.
4) People who have experienced at least one problem situation, with psychological distress, and GHQ above five.

In this way the effect of the three simultaneous indicators can be disentangled.

Apart from this, we will consider the group indicating mental distress in their diary. This group may contain members of each of the four previous groups.

Going to see the doctor

By combining the data from the health survey or the diary with the three-month registration of contacts with the general practitioner, we are able to describe the consulting behaviour of the four groups, created in the last paragraph.

In terms of the Goldberg & Huxley model, we are analyzing the permeability of the first filter: to what degree do mentally disturbed people seek help from a general practitioner and in which degree do they present psychological or social complaints to their general practitioner? In terms of need and demand: how do felt need and normative need relate to demand for psychosocial care?

Indicators from interview. Mental disorder is now operationalized from the view of the patient and of psychiatry by the three indicators "experience of psychosocial problems", "presence of problem situations" and "GHQ", which have been combined into four groups. For these indicators, the results are presented in table 3.6

Table 3.6
GP-contact and presentation of psychosocial complaints by patients with different needs

		Group 1[1]	Group 2	Group 3	Group4
N:		3721	2440	1745	987
GP visit	N:	1190	790	692	515
in 3-months:	%:	32%	32%	40%	52%
Average N of visits		1.95	2.05	2.2	2.9
Psychol. compl. (ICPC: P)	%:	2,9%	5,7%	10,7%	22,3%
Social compl. (ICPC: Z)	%:	2,9%	4,2%	4,8%	12,2%

[1] Group 1: No probl.situations, no psychological distress, GHQ < 5
2: At least one problem situation, no psychological distress, GHQ < 5
3: at least one problem situation, with psychological distress, GHQ < 5
4: at least one problem situation, with psychological distress, and GHQ ≥ 5

Table 3.6 should be read as follows: Group 1, people without any problem situation, who did not report any feeling of distress in the past two weeks and who scored negatively on the GHQ, consists of 3721 respondents. Of these 3721 persons, 1190 (32%) has contacted their general practitioner at least once during three months of registration. The average number of contacts of those who visited the general practitioner was 1.95. 2.9% of those who visited the general practitioner presented psychological complaints as reason for visit and also 2.9% presented social complaints, psychological and social complaints being those reasons for visit which were coded in ICPC-chapter P or Z.

Comparing the four groups, there seems to be little difference between groups 1 and group 2, who are similar in not having experienced psychosocial complaints and by scoring below GHQ-threshold, but differ from each other because of the problem situations existing for group 2.

There are marked differences however between these two groups together and each of the other groups. Consulting behaviour and presentation of psychosocial complaints increases from group 1/2 to group 3 and even further to group 4. If feelings of mental distress during the past period have been experienced, it makes a difference in terms of frequency of consulting a general practitioner and for the presentation of explicit psychological or social complaints and it makes a difference again, if those experiences are combined with a positive score on a screening list or not.

Something that is not reproduced in table 3.6, but is worthy of mention, is the help-seeking behaviour of the small group of patients who are GHQ-cases without reporting feelings of mental distress or problem situations. These patients show exactly the same help-seeking behaviour as the GHQ-cases who did report feelings of distress and problem situations.

The presence of problem situations alone does not influence medical consumption. People in these circumstances only present slightly more psychosocial complaints, when they visit the doctor. What matters, conversely, is the recent experience of emotional distress, especially when this is combined with an elevated GHQ-score. Therefore, in the remainder of this chapter we shall focus our attention on these two groups.

Although the probability of visiting a general practitioner is considerably higher for those who experience mental distress and/or are identified by the GHQ as probably mentally ill, we must stress the point that more than half of them did not contact their general practitioner at all during the three months of registration.

In the health interview, questions were asked about the date of the last general practitioner contact. This allows us to extrapolate the contact-rates for the different groups to longer periods, as is depicted in figure 3.4. This figure gives the cumulative proportion of patients who had at least one contact with the general practitioner within a certain time-interval. It is given for the three groups of patients we distinguished: those who felt no psychosocial need (and who accordingly were not attributed a normative need), those who felt a need but were not indicated as such by the GHQ, and those who both experienced mental distress and were considered probable cases of mental illness by the GHQ.

From this graph, it becomes clear that within a year the great majority of people, irrespective of their mental health status, had a contact with their general practitioner. However, those who combined feelings of mental distress with a positive GHQ generally had contact with the general practitioner within a considerably shorter time-interval than those without any problem.

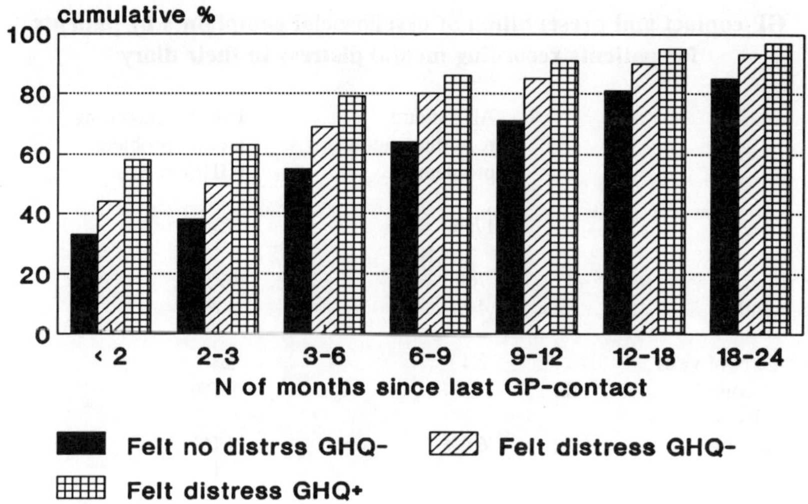

Figure 3.4 **Proportion of persons from different groups, having had a GP contact over various periods of time**

Although most mentally disturbed patients will see their general practitioner at some time, this certainly is no guarantee that they will contact him with psychosocial reasons for the visit. This is only true for less than one third of the group with probable psychopathology + experience of mental distress + problem situations, at least, if they do contact their general practitioner. The latter is true for about half of this group, so one sixth of this part of the population will take the initiative in discussing their mental problems with their general practitioner. When we restrict ourselves to those people who experienced mental distress in the previous weeks, but scored below GHQ-threshold, less than fifteen per cent of the visitors, being six per cent of that part of the population, are involved.

Indicators from diary. general practitioner-contact and problem-presentation of patients who indicated mental distress in their diary are presented in table 3.7.

Compared with the previous group of patients who responded affirmatively to questions about mental distress (Group 3 in table 3.6), these people who spontaneously recorded mental distress have visited their general practitioner more frequently, and have presented more psychological and social reasons for those visits.

Table 3.7
GP-contact and presentation of psychosocial complaints by patients for patients recording mental distress in their diary

		All patients recording mental problems	Patients recording mental problems (GHQ < 5)
N:		1754	1234
GP visit	N:	769	493
in 3-months:	%:	44%	40%
Average N of visits		2.4	2.3
Psychol. compl. (ICPC: P)	%:	15.7%	9.5%
Social compl. (ICPC: Z)	%:	6.8%	4.1%

However, group 3 in table 3.6 were patients who indicated emotional complaints but who were negative GHQ-cases. If only those persons who recorded mental problems in their diary and who scored below threshold on the GHQ are taken into account (last column in table 3.7), there is no difference in help-seeking behaviour between patients who affirm precoded questions about mental distress and patients who record their distress in a diary. Consequently, identifying a felt need by means of diary yields no other results for help-seeking than the interview method. For the sake of clarity, we will continue with the classification from table 3.6, based on health interview data.

Help seeking and patient characteristics

How is help seeking behaviour, given the presence of feelings of distress or probable psychopathology, related to patient characteristics? And how does health status interfere in this respect. As it appeared, in earlier analyses of our material, that patients, scoring high on the GHQ, also reported more chronic diseases, more acute complaints and a worse perception of health than people scoring low (Bensing and Verhaak 1994; see also Williams et al. 1986), multivariate analyses were carried out to assess the determinants for contact with the general practitioner within the three months of registration.

These analyses were carried out for three groups separately: patients without reported feelings of mental distress and a low GHQ-score, for patients with reported feelings and a low GHQ-score and for patients with reported feelings and a high GHQ-score (Group 1+2, Group 3, Group 4). A two-step analysis was carried out. In the first step all relevant background characteristics were included, in the second step health indicators were added. The tables with the logistic regression are given at the end of the chapter[8].

Figure 3.5 summarizes the results for these three subgroups as well.

Determinants[1]:	Group 1/2	Group 3		Group 4			
		BH[2]	AH	BH	AH	BH	AH
Sex	Male	–	–	–	–	–	–
	Female	+	+	+	+	+	+
Highest level of finished education:	Primary			+			
	Secondary			+			
	Higher			–			
Employment status	Housewife/man	+	+	+	+	+	+
	Unemployed			+	+		
	Incapacitated	+		+		+	+
	Retired	+	+	+	+	+	+
	Working/Student	–	–	–	–	–	–
Insurance	Public	+	+			+	+
	Private	–	–			–	–
Subjective health perception		0	+	0	+	0	
N of acute complaints		0	+	0	+	0	
N of chron. conditions		0	+	0		0	+

1 Age, and urbanization and marital status have been omitted, because no significant odds could be reported

2 BH: before introducing health indicators
AH: after introducing health indicators
+: odds in respect of other values significantly > 1
–: odds in respect of other values significantly < 1
0: determinant not included in analysis

Figure 3.5 Determinants contributing to the probability of help-seeking

In general, the following major trends can be distinguished. Women are more likely to visit their general practitioner in each condition, irrespective of their health status. The same is true for employment status: housewives and retired persons have a higher probability of a general practitioner-contact, before and after control for health status than people with paid employment. People who are out of work because of disability, visit their general practitioner more frequently, it is true, but this circumstance is a direct result of their inferior health status, subjectively (subjective health perception) as well as objectively (presence of chronic diseases). However, in case of high GHQ-score incapacitated persons remain frequent visitors, even after controlling for their health status.

Insurance status affects help seeking in the case of people without mental disturbance as well as in the case of people with a high GHQ-score, and it does so irrespective of health status. Educational level heightens the probability of help seeking in the case of persons who indicated feelings of mental disturbance during the interview, but again this is a contamination with health status (the less well-educated have worse health status than those with higher education).

Looking at the effect of health status on help seeking, it is remarkable that this effect is highest for patients without any mental disturbance and lowest for patients who experience feelings of mental distress paired with a high GHQ-score. In the first case all three health indicators add independently to the probability of a contact with the general practitioner, while in the latter case only the existence of chronic conditions exert an effect. A "normative need", as measured by the GHQ, has an effect on help seeking behaviour, independent of subjective health status.

Conclusions

Summary of results

In this chapter, mental disorder in the population has been considered from different points of view. About half of all the respondents of fifteen years and above found themselves recently in at least one psychosocial problem situation. In their own view, about thirty-five per cent observed on inquiry at least one psychosocial complaint and fifteen per cent spontaneously recorded such complaints during three weeks in a diary. According to an index of "normative need", in a psychiatric sense (General Health Questionnaire) thirteen per cent scored above threshold. Considering only these raw prevalences in the population, we can conclude that "felt need" exceeds "normative need" and that distress on inquiry is more frequent than spontaneously observed distress.

In whatever way disorder may have been operationalized, women, divorced people, disabled people and inhabitants of urbanized areas are always overrepresented, after controlling for other characteristics. Unemployed persons are at risk on three out of four measures: only according to their diary are they comparable to those employed.

Widows/widowers indicate more problem situations and have a higher probability on psychopathology, but they do not report more psychological distress, neither on inquiry nor in their diaries.

Older persons and the publicly-insured, on the other hand, report more feelings of distress but their burden of problem situations is not heavier, and their GHQ-score is not higher than those of younger or privately-insured persons. Education has a seemingly contradictory effect, as those with higher education report problem situations more frequently and record more feelings of distress in their diary than the less well-educated. Possibly a number of problem situations, having to do with relations and working situation, are typical for those with higher education, in employment, resulting also in a greater prevalence of "stress", the most popular complaint in the diary.

To summarize: women, people out of work, divorced people and large city inhabitants are more at risk for mental disorder from an expert point of view and they complain accordingly. Widows/widowers are at risk as well, but they do not complain. From the other hand, older people and publicly insured people are not more at risk, but are likely to complain, while better educated people define some of their living conditions as stressful but seem able to cope with it. A picture which is in line with the literature, discussed in chapter 1 and which partly nuances previous results (c.f. De Ridder 1988, Ypema and de Haan 1983, Vázquez Barquéro 1990, Williams et al. 1986).

There may be a lot of distress in the population, as subjective experience and from a professional psychiatric viewpoint as well, but only part of these people seek professional help immediately - i.e. within a restricted period of three months. In this respect, help seeking is more common among those who are professionally considered at great risk for severe psychopathology (GHQ+) than among those who report feelings of distress without scoring above GHQ-threshold. Furthermore, help-seeking among the former is less determined by their health status than help-seeking among those who are not a GHQ-case.

Some generalization is possible regarding patient characteristics which determine help-seeking, given mental distress of one sort or another, i.e.: women are more prone to visit a general practitioner than men and the unemployed more than the employed, even when health status is taken into account. There are some groups who have a higher probability of mental distress but who are not more likely to visit a general practitioner when experiencing distress or being a GHQ-case. We should mention the divorced, who are more likely to experience distress themselves and to score high on a professional index like the GHQ, but who do not visit their general practitioner, when belonging to such a group, more than married or single people. Older persons are more likely to report feelings of mental distress, but those of the elderly who actually report these feelings again do not visit their general practitioner more frequently than younger people reporting distress. Widows/widowers are more at risk of psychopathology, but those who are actually detected by the GHQ will not see the general practitioner more often than married, single or divorced people.

Results compared with other research

A comparison with other findings is easiest for the GHQ findings, because this instrument is most frequently cited in literature. We report a point prevalence of "GHQ-caseness" of 125/1000. Goldberg and Huxley (1980) depart from a point-prevalence of 184/1000. In our introduction we presented other point-prevalences of an even higher level, ranging from 185/1000 to 234/1000. Goldberg and Huxley also cite Finlay-Jones and Burvill, 1977 who found 120/1000.

A possible explanation of our relatively low figure may be the conditions under which the GHQ has been assessed. In contrast with other research, in our survey the GHQ was hidden in a two-hour interview between a large set of questionnaires and questions covering the total field of health experience, health services use, opinions and attitudes. The respondents' attention was not directed at mental health at all. This may have resulted in a slighter probability of "complaining on request".[9]

Another methodological point to be made has to do with the (possible) lack of concurrence in time between completion of the GHQ and other questionnaires and contact with the general practitioner. Therefore, analyses of determinants of a doctor-patient contact have been repeated with only those patients who consulted their doctor within three weeks of the interview. The results were exactly the same (Verhaak, in press).

86% of those who were positive on the GHQ indicated a contact with their general practitioner during a one-year period. This figure is comparable with other results regarding Goldberg and Huxley's first filter: Goldberg and Huxley themselves estimate this proportion as being 92%, Giel, Koeter and Ormel (1990), replicating the Goldberg and Huxley figures in their own research arrive at 74%.

Although our estimate of psychopathology, based on the GHQ, is lower than most other studies, the relationships found are comparable with other studies, mentioned in the introduction to this chapter. All investigators (Finlay-Jones and Burvill 1977, Vasquez-Barquero et al. 1990, Williams et al. 1986) report an overrepresentation of women, divorced and unemployed people among the GHQ-cases.

Another agreement with other research is found in the result that many people experience psychosocial problems every once in a while, but severe psychopathology is probable among only a part of them. On the other hand, most people who suffer probably from psychopathology experience feelings of distress, too (c.f. Hodiamont et al. 1987).

Epilogue

This chapter dealt with the first two research questions: how do felt needs of patients relate to their normative needs and what consequences have these needs for help-seeking behaviour.
Experience of problem situations and feelings of distress are very common phenomena. A subsample of this large group of persons is selected by an instrument like the GHQ, and are thus considered, from a psychiatric point of view, as being probably severely mentally ill. As this subsample is a selection of the larger group of distressed persons, the characteristics of the persons in this selection are the same as those in the larger group, but not all characteristics of the larger group are found in the GHQ-group.

Thus, the professional selects people who are distressed according to their own experience as well. In other words, there is a kind of agreement between GHQ/professional viewpoint on the one hand, and the lay-judgement/subjective experience on the other hand. The interesting point is what happens where there is no such agreement between felt need and normative need. One kind of lack of agreement is shown by those persons who manifest moments of mental distress, without being selected by the GHQ. How are they coping with their problems? They visit their doctor less frequently than those, selected by the GHQ, and put forward less demands for psychological or social complaints. They seem to manage better without medical help than the GHQ-cases. The other failure to agreement is shown by those whose GHQ-score points to a normative need while they do not report experiences of mental distress. Although they seem to deny the expert evaluation they show help-seeking behaviour comparable with GHQ cases who experienced feelings of mental distress as well.

Another area of tension, and the essential theme of this book, is the possible discrepancy between normative and felt need at the one hand and demand for help at the other. In this respect we should point to the majority of those who experience distress (all or not confirmed by the GHQ) but who do not look for professional help (for example those 48% of the GHQ-cases who did not visit a doctor during the three month registration and 60% of those who experienced feelings of distress without being a GHQ case). Many of these seem to find other solutions than medical care for their mental disorder. At least, our data suggest that there are no serious limitations to the access of care. Because, less well-educated people, people from rural areas or publicly insured persons have either better or equal chances for seeking medical care in case of mental disorder (be it a felt need or a need according to professional standards).

Of course, going to see the doctor is not the same as demanding help for mental disorder. The way this is determined is the main issue in the next chapter.

Notes

1. The range indicates differences between the three sites, considered at that moment. The increase of prevalence with increasing period of reference is visible in next figure:

DSM-diagnosis during:	Prevalence range (N/1000 respondents)
previous two weeks:	72 - 86
previous month:	82 - 106
previous half year:	116 - 132
previous year:	137 - 152
lifelong:	230 - 252

(Source: Myers et al., 1984)

2. SC Newman and RC Bland report in the Canadian Study of Health and Aging a strong relationship between stress events and social problems on the one hand and DIS-cases on the other hand. (Newman SC and Bland RC, a community survey in Edmonton, Canada, paper presented at "Epidemiology in psychiatry and mental health", congress of the International Federation of Psychiatric Epidemiology, Lisbon, 14 - 17 April, 1993.

3. Some items from the list of physical problems, for instance headache or bowel movement, are classified as "physical" but might have a psychosocial connotation. It remains debatable whether those items should be included in the experience of psychological symptoms.
   One reason for not including them has to do with our research questions. We want to know to what extent feelings of psychological distress are prevalent in the population and produce an effect on medical consumption.
   A second reason for limiting ourselves to the psychosocial items is found in our data. During the registration of doctor-patient contacts, each reason for encounter was assessed by the GP on a 5-point-scale for the psychosocial character of the reason for visit. The following table presents the average score given by GPs when complaints from the check-list were actually presented.

Table 3.8
Assessment of complaints by GP on a 5-point-scale

Psychological complaints:					
	N:	mean		N:	mean
Nervous	2185	4.5	Sleeplessness	1233	4.1
Easily agitated/ Aggressive feelings	384	3.9	Listlessness	1414	4.5
Family problems	214	4.8			
Physical complaints:					
Headache	5847	2.4	Tiredness	6311	2.6
Stuffy nose	1465	1.3	Cough	13894	1.2
Back complaints	8682	1.7	Neck/shoulder	3009	1.2
Sore throat	5464	1.4	Dizziness	3056	2.4
Excessive perspiration	223	2.3	Hearing difficulty	245	1.2
Tightness in the chest	3556	1.6	Oppressed in chest	265	2.1
Abdominal cramp	6000	2.2	Bowel Movement	265	1.9
Ringing in the ears	397	1.7	Heartburn	337	1.7
Stomachache	2062	2.2	Heart palpitations	679	2.7
Nausea	758	2.1	Increase in weight	118	2.7
Swollen ankles	524	1.2	Diarrhoea	1548	1.3
Menstrual pain	808	1.6	Fever	3661	1.2
Earache	3989	1.2	Toothache	169	1.3
Vomiting	988	1.5	Incontinence	349	1.7
Nose bleeding	354	1.2	Eating problem	133	2.4
Burning sensation on urination	1261	1.2			

Items characterized as psychosocial have an average rating above four, while physical items have a range from 1.2 to 2.7. Furthermore, it can be observed that the scores between 1.2 and 2.7 are distributed rather equally, then there is a gap between 2.7 and 4.1.

4.

Table 3.9
Logistic regression on the experience of psychosocial complaints as reported during the health interview

Determinant:	B	sign.	odds	in respect of:
Sex				female
- male	-.54	.000	.58	
Age	.01	.000	1.01	
Insurance				public
- private	-.16	.000	.85	
Employment status				employed
- housewife/man	.09	n.s	-	
- unemployed	.31	.024	1.37	
- incapacitated	1.01	.000	2.77	
- retired	-.04	n.s	-	
Marital status				unmarried
- married	-.18	.002	.83	
- divorced	.61	.000	1.84	
- widows/widowers	.20	n.s	-	
Urbanization				3 large cities
- rural	-.54	.000	.58	
- suburban	-.45	.000	.64	
- urban	-.17	n.s	-	

The dependent variable in this analysis was the probability that someone would experience at least one psychosocial complaint during the previous two weeks. The dichotomy is between no complaints and one complaint or more. We have made an analysis to see if the relationships would change if the criterion (any psychosocial complaint) were accentuated, for instance to the dichotomy zero or one complaint versus two or more complaints. With a sharpened criterion, most of the effects remain the same. When we discriminate between persons with two complaints or less versus three and more, there is no longer any difference between married and unmarried people, and when switching from three complaints or fewer to four or more, the age-effect disappears.

5.

Table 3.10
Logistic regression on the experience of psychosocial complaints as registered in the health diary

Determinant:	B	sign.	odds	in respect of:
Sex				female
- male	-.755	.000	.47	
Employment status				employed
- housewife/man	.09	n.s	-	
- unemployed	-.42	.050	.65	
- incapacitated	.41	.010	1.50	
- retired	-.23	.025	.79	
Marital status				unmarried
- married	-.04	n.s	-	
- divorced	.44	.002	1.55	
- widows/widowers	.06	n.s	-	
Urbanization				3 large cities
- rural	-.58	.000	.56	
- suburban	-.50	.000	.61	
- urban	-.25	.045	.77	
Education				Higher education
- primary	-.96	.000	.38	
- secondary	-.49	.000	.61	

6.

Table 3.11
Logistic regression on the existence of problematic situations

Determinant:	B	sign.	odds	in respect of:
Sex				female
- male	-.19	.000	.83	
Employment status				employed
- housewife/man	.09	n.s	-	
- unemployed	.79	.000	2.20	
- incapacitated	.53	.000	1.70	
- retired	-.19	.005	.83	
Marital status				unmarried
- married	-.03	n.s	-	
- divorced	.84	.000	2.31	
- widows/widowers	.24	.021	1.27	
Urbanization				3 large cities
- rural	-.60	.000	.55	
- suburban	-.45	.000	.64	
- urban	-.27	.013	.77	
Education				Higher education
- primary	-.96	.000	.38	
- secondary	-.49	.000	.61	

7.

Table 3.12

Logistic regression on a score ≥ 5 on the GHQ

Determinant:	B	sign.	odds	in respect of:
Sex				female
- male	-.57	.000	.57	
Employment status				employed
- housewife/man	.16	n.s	-	
- unemployed	.53	.003	1.71	
- incapacitated	1.02	.000	2.77	
- retired	-.08	n.s	-	
Marital status				unmarried
- married	-.07	n.s	-	
- divorced	.73	.000	2.08	
- widows/widowers	.36	.008	1.44	
Urbanization				3 large cities
- rural	-.57	.000	.56	
- suburban	-.38	.002	.68	
- urban	-.27	.042	.76	

8. **Table 3.13**

Predicting the probability of visiting a GP from patient characteristics and their health status for patients without mental disturbance

	Before adding health			After adding health			
Determinant:	B	sign.	odds	B	sign.	odds	in respect of
Insurance							public
- private	-.21	.000	.81	-.43	.003	.65	
Sex							female
- male	-.28	.000	.76	-.33	.012	.72	
Employment status							employed
- housewife/man	.40	.000	1.50	.64	.000	1.89	
- unemployed	.02	n.s	-	1.07	.002	2.92	
- incapacitated	.71	.000	2.04	.49	n.s	1.63	
- retired	1.25	.000	3.48	1.17	.000	3.23	
N of acute complaints				.11	.000	1.12	
N of chronic conditions	-	-	-	.12	.003	1.13	
Subjective health perception				.32	.000	1.38	

Table 3.14

Predicting the probability of visiting a GP from patient characteristics and their health status for patients with feelings of mental disturbance but scoring below GHQ-threshold.

	Before adding health			After adding health			
Determinant:	B	sign.	odds	B	sign.	odds	in respect of
Education							higher
- only primary	.51	.006	1.66	-	n.s	-	
- secondary	.38	.042	1.47	-	n.s	-	
Sex							female
- male	-.33	.004	.72	-.30	.008	.74	
Employment status							employed
- housewife/man	.66	.000	1.94	.70	.000	2.01	
- unemployed	1.05	.000	2.87	1.04	.001	2.82	
- incapacitated	.61	.020	1.84	-	n.s	-	
- retired	1.84	.000	6.27	.97	.000	2.62	
N of acute complaints	-	-	-	.14	.003	1.15	
N of chronic conditions	-	-	-	-	n.s	-	
Subjective health perception	-	-	-	.36	.000	1.44	

Table 3.15
Predicting the probability of visiting a GP from patient characteristics and their health status for patients with feelings of mental disturbance and scoring above GHQ-threshold.

	Before adding health			After adding health			
Determinant:	B	sign.	odds	B	sign.	odds	in respect of
Insurance							compulsory
- private	-.56	.002	.57	-.53	.004	.59	
Sex							fcmalc
- male	-.36	.036	.70	-.36	.04	.70	
Employment status							employed
- housewife/man	.78	.000	2.19	.68	.001	1.98	
- unemployed	.10	n.s.	1.10	.09	n.s.	1.09	
- incapacitated	1.02	.000	2.78	.89	.002	2.44	
- retired	.95	.000	2.59	.78	.000	2.19	
N of acute complaints	-	-	-	-	n.s.	-	
N of chronic conditions	-	-	-	.12	.013	1.13	
Subjective health perception	-	-	-	-	n.s.	-	

9. This explanation is in line with the finding that a GHQ-12, administered without further items or questionnaires, needs a higher cut-off point to reach comparable test characteristics with a GHQ-12 nested within a GHQ-60 (personal communication from B.v.Hemert).

4 Mental disorder in general practice: From complaint to diagnosis

Introduction

In chapter 3, mental disorder in the population has been described. In general, three relevant levels of mental disorder could be distinguished: people who do not experience any feelings of mental disorder and who are not indicated by the GHQ as being probably disturbed, people who actually experience such feelings without scoring above GHQ-threshold, and people who both experience mental disorder and are identified by the GHQ as well. The second group represents those who feel in need, the third group the people who feel in need and are considered professionally in need as well. A certain number from each group consulted their general practitioner during the research period of three months. We continue our analyses with the complaints presented by these patients and the diagnoses attached to them by the general practitioner. It is here that demand for help comes into the picture.

Before returning to our study population, we shall first summarize the current findings in literature concerning mental disorder among people contacting primary health care facilities. We distinguish between two kinds of assessment: the standardized approach which was introduced in chapter 1 by means of psychiatric screening-lists or standardized clinical interviews at the one hand, and assessments by the general practitioner, be it a diagnosis or a precoded assessment on the other hand. The former approach captures the "normative need" from the psychiatric viewpoint while the latter can be considered as the "normative need" from the viewpoint of the general practitioner.

Investigator	Prev/1000	♂ : ♀	Details
Bellantuono et al. 1987 (Italy)	460	1:1	N = 90 GHQ-30 with cut-off point at 5/6
Goldberg, Kay and Thompson 1976 (UK)	297	1:1.2	N = 365
Goldberg and Bridges 1987 (UK)	452		N = 590
Hoeper et al. 1979 (USA)	300		N = 1072
Kessler et al. 1985 (USA)	278		N = 1452
v. Limbeek et al. 1994 (The Netherlands)	377		N = 2417
v d Meer 1994 (The Netherlands)	460		N = 2149
Skuse en Williams 1984 (UK)	390		N = 272 "True prevalence" after validating the GHQ was 340

Figure 4.1 Prevalence rates of mental disorder per 1000 patients visiting a GP; based on direct assessment by the GHQ (cut-off point at 4/5, unless otherwise indicated)

A review of psychiatric research in general practice

The psychiatric point of view

GHQ-research In many studies focusing on mental disorder in primary care settings, the GHQ is administered among patients consulting their general practitioners. The GHQ score is often compared with a general practitioner-assessment of the psychiatric character of the symptoms presented. Figure 4.1 shows the prevalence of psychiatric morbidity, measured in GHQ-studies. According to the GHQ, about thirty to fifty per cent of all those attending a general practitioner's-practice have a high probability of serious mental distress at the time of visit. This prevalence is clearly higher than the prevalence of GHQ-cases in population studies, reported in figure

3.1, which was to be expected. As far as characteristics of patients are reported, it is remarkable that the differences between sexes have almost disappeared.

The standardized psychiatric interview Figure 4.2 presents an overview of studies in which the prevalence of mental disorder has been assessed by means of complete standardized psychiatric interviews in primary care settings. As has been remarked earlier, these interviews result in a smaller number false positives than screening questionnaires and thus yield lower, more reliable prevalence rates.

Nevertheless we can conclude from figure 4.2 that for twenty to almost thirty-five per cent of the patients who visit a general practitioner a current DIS-problem or DSM-III diagnosis can still be established. The Groningen study (Wilmink 1990) is an exception with about ten per cent diagnoses, resulting from the PSE. Goldberg and Bridges, however, using the same interview, generated more than three times as many PSE diagnoses. Differences between men and women are hardly reported.

Investigator	Prev/1000	♂ : ♀	Details
Bellantuono et al. 1987 (Italy)	388		N = 90 CIS[1]
Goldberg and Bridges 1987 (UK)	331		(N=283) DSM-III
	267		PSE/ID-Catego
Hoeper et al. 1979 (USA)	276		(N = 247) SADS-L
Kessler et al. 1987 (USA)	±180- ±260	1:1.1	(N = ± 3000 - 5000) Current DIS in 5 areas in ECA-survey[2]
v. Limbeek et al. 1994 (The Netherlands)	233		Current DIS (N = 639)
Schulberg et al. 1985 (USA)	312		(N = 294) Current DIS
Wilkinson en Barczak 1988 (UK)	330		(N = 100) DSM-III diagnosis
Wilmink 1989 (NL)	105	1:1	N = 297 PSE

Figure 4.2 Prevalence rates of mental disorder per 1000 patients visiting a GP; based on standardized psychiatric interviews

Diagnoses of mental disorder made by general practitioners

In a number of studies general practitioners have been requested to assess the possible psychosocial character of complaints, presented to them, on precoded scales. This procedure has for the first time been reported by Crombie (1963), who presented the results of ten general practitioners, based on 1223 assessments. Illnesses of 52% of consecutive contacts with new patients were rated as "(nearly) all organic)", 21% as "mainly organic but with some abnormal emotional content", 13% as "emotional and organic in equal proportion", 6% as "mainly emotional but with some organic content" and 8% as "(nearly) all emotional".

	1)	2)	3)	4)	5)	6)
N:	590	553	272	256	227	990
Entirely physical illness	74%	58%	59%	60%	48%	53%
Physical illness with secondary psychiatric illness	7%	13%	26%	10%	31%	18%
Unrelated physical and psychiatric illness	5%	7%	5%	20%	6%	
Psychiatric illness with somatic symptoms	9%	12%	3%	8%	2%	13%
Entirely psychiatric illness	5%	10%	6%	4%	13%	

1) Goldberg and Bridges 1987
2) Goldberg and Blackwell 1970
3) Skuse and Williams 1984
4) Wilkinson and Markus 1989
5) Wright and Perini 1987
6) Verhaak 1986

Figure 4.3 Assessment by GP according to Goldberg's categories[3]

About ten years after, Goldberg and Blackwell (1970) used a comparable scale which has been used since - sometimes in slightly adapted versions - in a number of studies.

In figure 4.3 the results of a number of such studies have been reproduced. It can be seen that a general practitioner, if not restricted by diagnostic categories, generally considers thirty to more than forty per cent of the problems he encounters as being not strictly of a physical nature. At the other end of the continuum it can be seen that this does not mean for the general practitioner that all these problems are entirely psychiatric; no more than about ten per cent of all general practitioner assessments result in such a definition. In many more cases, however, mental or psychiatric problems play a role in one way or another without them being psychiatric illnesses in a strict sense.

Investigator	Prev/1000	♂ : ♀	Definition
Goldberg, Kay en Thompson (1976) (UK) (N = 365)	367 (point)	1:1.3	"Significant degree of psychiatric disturbance"
Huygen et al. 1984 (NL) (N = 11880)	100 (year)	1:1.3 (new) 1:1.4 (chron)	Diagnosis "Nervous-function complaint" on E-list
Jencks 1985 (USA) (N = 16576)	56 (year)		ICD-9 mental diagnosis*
Lamberts en Hartman 1982 (NL) (N = 16863)	140 (year)	♀ > ♂	ICPHPPC-2 chapter V
Lamberts 1991 (NL) (N = 40976)	158 (year)	♀ > ♂	ICPC: Chapter P (Psychological)
	124 (year)	♀ > ♂	ICPC: Chapter Z (Social)
Marks, Goldberg en Hillier 1979 (UK) (N = 4098)	311 (point)	♀ > ♂	GP's judgment: conspicuous psychiatric morbidity
Swartling et al. 1987 (Sweden) (N = 3205 resp. 2724)	173 resp. 177 (point)	1:4	"psychiatric symptoms/psycho-social problems"**
Third National Study ('81-'82)(UK)	109 (year)	1:2	Mental Disorder (E-list)
Wilmink (1989) (NL) (N = 1994)	257 (point)	1:1	"Mental Health Prob. symptoms coming from emotional conflict or stress-situation"

* Diagnoses made by internists, family practitioners and GPs

** Diagnoses made by doctors in training, GPs and specialists in health centre

Figure 4.4 Prevalence of mental disorder, as diagnosed by GPs

Figure 4.4 summarizes those studies in which general practitioners categorized their diagnosis or assessment of the problem in another way. Those studies in which only a global assessment is given by the general practitioner yield higher prevalences of mental disorder than the ones in which the general practitioner is forced to categorize his diagnosis into the International Classification of Diseases (ICD), International Classification of Health Problems in Primary Care (ICHPPC-2), E-list or International Classification of Primary Care (ICPC). Wilmink, Goldberg et al. and Marks et al., using the first approach, report twenty-five to thirty five per cent of all patients consulting being mentally ill. The family practice oriented diagnostic systems, like ICHPPC-2 and E-list remain under fifteen per cent and when only strict psychiatric categories are used (ICD), no more than five per cent of psychiatric cases are reported.

In contrast to results of standardized instruments, general practitioners report an overrepresentation of women among the identified cases. Those diagnoses are most common among the middle aged. Goldberg and Huxley also report higher rates of general practitioners' diagnoses for divorced, widows/widowers and unemployed patients (Goldberg and Huxley 1980). They have pointed to the possibility that general practitioners overestimate the prevalence of mental disorder within certain groups of patients, such like middle-aged women, whose complaints are easily and stereotypically labelled as "psychological". Among such groups many "false positives" are found, while groups with a contrary stereotype (young males) contain a lot of "false negatives". The same phenomenon has been reported by Bensing and Beerendonk (1990).

An important feature of diagnoses of mental disorder made by general practitioners is the so called "inter-doctor variation". Marks, Goldberg and Hillier (1979) reported considerable differences between general practitioner's tendency to label patients' symptoms as "psychiatric". Their average 311/1000, given in figure 4.4, had a range from 30/1000 to 770/1000. Goldberg and Huxley (1980) called this tendency the ***bias*** of the general practitioner and found this bias to be related to doctor's shown interest and concern during consultations, to asking questions of a psychiatric nature and doctor's interest in psychiatry.

In an earlier study of our own, we found the same variation between doctors. Our average 53% assessments "entirely physical illness" in figure 4.3 has a range from 24% to 83%. In this study, we were able to characterize the consulting style of doctors with a high rate of psychosocial diagnoses as being more patient-centered (which concept included "shown interest" and "concern", mentioned by Goldberg and Huxley). These doctors were also more concerned with psychogenic factors in illness (Verhaak 1986).

Related to the ***bias*** of general practitioners are two other concepts, introduced by Goldberg: the ***accuracy*** of the general practitioner and the *identification index*. In contradistinction to the bias, the latter two must be related to some kind of gold standard, as they express the ability of a general practitioner to recognize "real" cases correctly. The identification index is the proportion "real" cases identified by the general practitioner. The accuracy is the agreement between a general practitioner's assessment and a gold standard. Identification index is directed at the proportion "true positives" while the accuracy takes into account the proportion "false positives" as well. As the identification index increases with the number of identified "cases", it is associated with a general practitioner's bias. If a general practitioner considers each patient as a case of mental disorder, he undoubtedly has not missed any case, but many patients will have been labelled mentally ill unjustified. Identification index, thus, is associated with the same doctor-characteristics as bias. Accuracy was especially related to an interview style of the general practitioner which was characterized as "directive interviewer with accurate concepts" as well as to clinical competence.

We can summarize this brief overview of the existing literature as follows: In general prevalence of mental disorder among people who have passed Goldberg and Huxley's first filter is higher than in the population. Global assessments or screening-instruments yield higher prevalences than diagnostic categories and standardized interviews. From a psychiatric point of view, the prevalence of mental disorder is higher than seen by a general practitioner. Between general practitioners there are considerable differences in their tendency to make psychosocial diagnoses as well as in their ability to detect probable cases accurately. We will now turn to our own results in these respects.

Input: complaints presented by the patient (demand)

3950 respondents who visited their general practitioner during the three-month registration presented 8734 reasons for encounter (RFE). The distribution of these RFE's over the eighteen chapters of ICPC is presented in figure 4.5.

In this average group of patients, complaints regarding the musculo-skeletal system are most common. Almost one quarter of all complaints presented belong to this category. These are followed by general complaints (general weakness, infections not else classifiable, pain, fever), complaints concerning the respiratory system, the skin and the digestive system. Five per cent of all complaints are classified within the category "Psychological" and two per cent within the category "Social". Given our research questions, we will concentrate on the latter two categories.

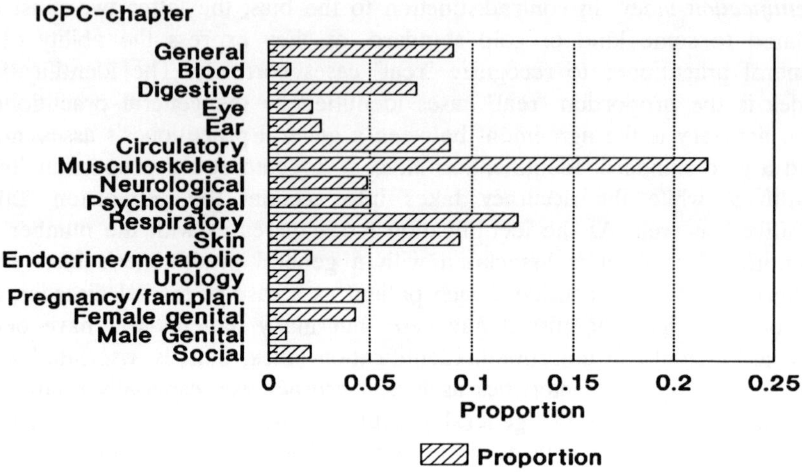

Figure 4.5 Distribution of reasons for encounter over 18 ICPC-chapters

Table 4.1 gives the ten psychological and social complaints most frequently presented.

Anxiety and depression are the most common psychosocial complaints. A substantial number of patients also present an already established diagnosis, e.g.: "neurotic depression" as reason for the present visit.

Table 4.1
Top-ten of psychosocial complaints, presented in general practice (N/10,000)

		N/10,000
1)	Anxiety	98
2)	Feelings of depression	56
3)	Sleep disturbance	47
4)	Acute stress reaction	36
5)	Problems re:working situation	33
6)	Partner problems	22
7)	Restless, agitated	20
8)	Memory problems	14
9)	Neurotic depression	14
10)	Smoking addiction	11

Not in the top-ten, as they are no "complaints" in a strict sense, but nevertheless rather common, are requests for medication, further investigation or referral as a reason for consulting the general practitioner. For instance, 78 out of 10,000 RFE's are requests for psychofarmaca, making it the second most important psychological RFE.

Complaints according to level of distress

Again, patients have been divided in three groups; those who did not experience psychological distress nor had an elevated GHQ-score, those who actually experienced such feelings but did not score above GHQ-threshold and the group of patients who combined feelings of mental distress with an elevated GHQ.

Figure 4.6 shows the percentages of complaints falling in several ICPC-chapters, only for those instances where substantial differences between the three groups could be noticed.

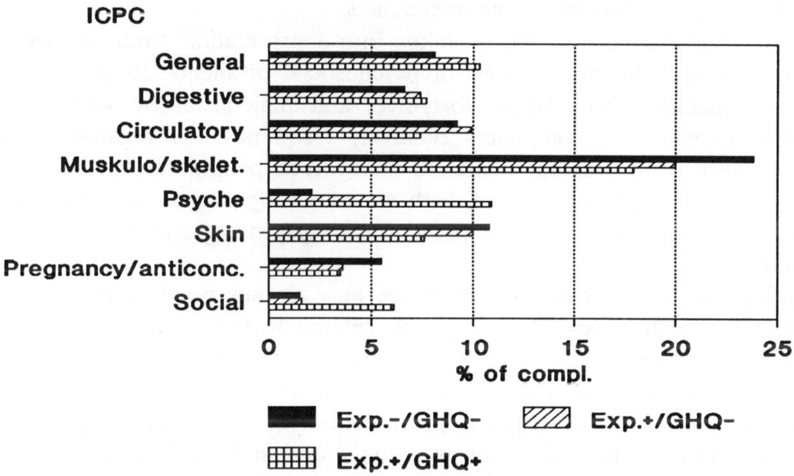

Figure 4.6 Distribution of RFE over ICPC-chapters for three categories of patients with different degrees of mental distress

As was to be expected, the contribution of psychological complaints increases considerably when patients had experienced feelings of mental distress in the recent past and increased again when patients scored high on the GHQ. This had already been pointed out in the previous chapter (table 3.6). Increases are also observed for the ICPC-chapters "General", "Digestive" and "Social". On the contrary, the relative share of disorders of the Musculo/Skeletal system, the Circulatory system, Skin and Pregnancy decreases.

The ranking of the most frequently presented psychosocial complaints (table 4.1) remains largely the same for the different groups, but as was to be expected, the prevalences increases, with patients who did not experience any feelings of distress at the lowest level and patients who scored positively on the GHQ on the highest. For anxiety, depression, disturbed sleep and feelings of restlessness, the increase is linear. For example, 36 out of 10,000 patients without any distress presented complaints of anxiety. This figure is 120/10,000 for patients who experienced feelings of distress without being a GHQ-case and 218/10,000 for GHQ-cases. Complaints regarding working conditions, acute stress or partner-problems are for the both first groups on an equal -low- level, and are elevated for the GHQ+-group only.

Presentation of psychosocial complaints and patient-characteristics

Table 4.2 summarizes the relationship between presentation of psychosocial problems and several patient characteristics.

Of all characteristics which are taken into consideration, three are clearly associated with the presentation of psychosocial problems. Regarding age, adults, especially those below forty-five, and patients above seventy-five, present psychosocial complaints relatively frequently. As regards marital status, there is an overrepresentation of divorced people among those with psychosocial complaints. At last, with an increasing degree of urbanization patients are more inclined to present with psychological or social complaints.

Anticipating the discussion section, we may already point to the discrepancy between the many characteristics, related to the experience of problems and the probability of psychopathology (female, widows/widowers, older, publicly-insured, unemployed, large cities) and the lack of such relationships with the explicit presentation of psychosocial problems. Perhaps, part of the explanation must be found in a tendency to somatize mental disorder. This aspect is one of the themes of the following subchapter.

Table 4.2
Proportion of visitors who reported psychological and social complaints, with different background characteristics

		N[1]	% of psychol. complaints	X^2	% of social complaints	X^2
Sex	Male	3408	5.2%	3.2(ns)	2.6%	.04 (ns)
	Female	5326	6.1%		2.6%	
Age	15-24	1312	3.3%	35.7*	1.5%	16.8**
	25-44	3130	6.5%		3.1%	
	45-64	2548	6.2%		2.4%	
	65-74	1134	4.0%		2.0%	
	75+	610	8.7%		4.1%	
Marital status	Married	5650	5.8%	23.9*	2.5%	8.9***
	Divorced	363	11.3%		4.1%	
	Widows/widowers	849	5.9%		3.7%	
	Unmarried	1872	4.8%		2.1%	
Highest level of education completed	Only primary school	3062	5.3%	8.8(ns)	2.1%	8.2 (ns)
	Techn./Voc.Training 12-16 yrs	2122	6.5%		3.3%	
	Lower general second. education	1087	5.3%		2.9%	
	Techn./Voc Training 16-18 yrs	897	6.9%		2.3%	
	Higher general second. education	406	5.9%		2.7%	
	Techn./Voc. Tr. 18+	565	5.7%		2.8%	
	University	102	2.0%		3.9%	
Employment status	Student/Conscript	564	3.2%	6.2(ns)	1.6%	6.2 (ns)
	Housewife/man	1605	5.5%		2.1%	
	Unemployed	221	2.3%		3.2%	
	Incapacitated	464	6.0%		2.2%	
	Retired	1918	5.6%		2.7%	
	Employed	3023	6.5%		2.9%	
Insurance	Public	6326	6.0%	2.2(ns)	2.4%	.29 (ns)
	Private	2369	5.2%		2.7%	
Urbanization	Rural	3507	4.8%	12.7**	2.3%	7.4 (ns)
	Suburban	3303	6.1%		2.6%	
	Urban	1545	7.2%		2.8%	
	3 large cities	436	5.0%		4.4%	

* $p < .0001$ ** $p < .01$ *** $p < .05$

[1] N indicates the total number of RFE's of persons in the considered category

Transformation: from complaint to diagnosis

Complaints and diagnoses compared

Patients present complaints and problems, which are categorized within the ICPC-classification system. After further history-taking and diagnostic examinations the general practitioner establishes a diagnosis, which has been classified within ICPC too. In most cases, the diagnosis is specified within a diagnostic category, distinct from the symptom category in which the complaint has been classified, unless a symptom-diagnosis has been given. And neither is it necessary for the complaint and diagnosis to be classified within the same chapter. For instance, the complaint "headache", falling within ICPC-chapter "Neurology", may lead to a diagnosis "Hypertension", a diagnosis from chapter "Circulatory".

Table 4.3 shows that some complaints are rather frequently associated with diagnoses in the same ICPC-chapter, for example 86% of the complaints within the chapter "Pregnancy" are diagnosed within the same chapter. On the other hand, less than one third of the complaints, classified within the chapter "Neurology" are diagnosed within that chapter.

In this way, psychological complaints are diagnosed within the chapter "Psyche" in almost three quarter of all cases. On the other hand, more than ten per cent of the complaints within the chapters "General", "Digestive", "Neurology" and "Social", are also fitted with a diagnostic label from the chapter "Psyche".

A switch from non-psychosocial complaints to a psychosocial diagnosis is relatively often observed for unmarried persons, women, the younger age categories and people with paid employment. This is remarkable, in that sense, that most of these characteristics are not indicating a larger risk for mental disorder in general, as we saw in the previous chapter. Only the fact that somatic complaints of women are relatively often translated in a psychological diagnosis fits within that picture, as well as within a stereotype general practitioners might have, according to the literature (see fig. 4.4).

The picture, sketched in table 4.3, almost remains the same when we concentrate on those persons who have experienced mental distress in the recent past. However, within the subgroup of those who are also indicated by the GHQ as probable cases of mental disorder, a larger proportion of complaints from the chapters "General" (21%), "Blood" (23%), "Digestive" (12%), "Eye" (10%), "Musculo/skeletal" (10%), "Neurology" (22%) and "Social" (37%) are given with a psychological diagnosis. From this finding, we might conclude that a certain sensitivity for mental disorder, as indicated by the GHQ, is present among general practitioners. This sensitivity is further investigated in the next subchapter.

Table 4.3
Relationship between ICPC-chapter of complaint and diagnosis

Complaint (chapter)	Proportion diagnosis within same chapter used	Frequently alternatives
General	23%	Musculo/skelet. (16%)
		Psyche (11%)
		Respiratory (13%)
Blood	51%	General (15%)
Digestive	62%	Psyche (11%)
Eye	77%	
Ear	79%	
Circulatory	76%	
Musculo/skeletal	59%	Skin (16%)
Neurology	29%	Musculo/skeletal (10%)
		Psyche (18%)
		Respiratory (14%)
Psyche	72%	Social (9%)
Respiratory	78%	
Skin	76%	
Endocrinology	71%	
Urology	63%	
Pregnancy/Anticonception	86%	
Gynaecology	73%	
Urology	64%	Neurology (12%)
Social	48%	Psyche (26%)

Psychosocial assessment by the general practitioner

Except by a diagnosis within ICPC-chapters "Psyche" or "Social", general practitioners had another way for expressing their psychosocial assessment of patient and complaint. As explained in chapter 2, each diagnosis was accompanied by a five-point scale assessment of the possible role of psychosocial factors. In this way, a diagnosis within the chapter "Musculoskeletal", for example "low backache", could be provided with an assessment "more psychological than somatic".

The distribution of these assessments over all diagnoses is given in table 4.4.

Table 4.4
Assessment of diagnoses by the GP on 5-point scale "somatic-psychosocial"

Assessment	% of all diagnoses
Purely somatic	68.3%
More somatic than psychosocial	9.6%
As much somatic as psychosocial	10.5%
More psychosocial than somatic	3.7%
Purely psychosocial	7.9%

Figure 4.7 illustrates how these assessments are distributed over the several ICPC-chapters.

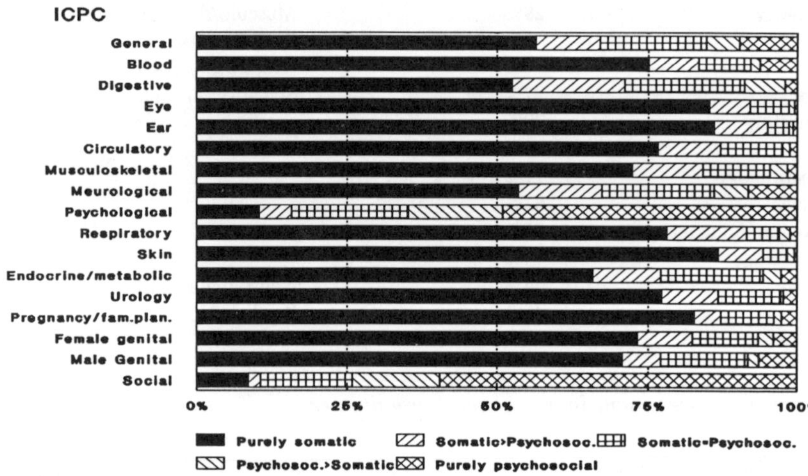

Figure 4.7 Assessment "somatic-psychosocial" for diagnoses on different ICPC-chapters

From table 4.4 and figure 4.7 it becomes clear that the number of recognized psychosocial problems in general practice exceeds the number of formal diagnoses within ICPC-chapters "Psychological" and "Social", which constitute about ten per cent of all diagnoses. In particular diagnoses within the chapters "General", "Digestive" and "Neurology" are relatively often considered as "not purely somatic". These are the same chapters from which complaints are relatively often "translated" into a psychological diagnosis (table 4.3).

On the contrary, the general practitioner considers the role of psychosocial factors rather limited with diagnoses in the chapters "Eye" (14.8% not entirely somatic), "Ear" (14%), Skin (13.2%) and "Pregnancy/anti-conception" (17.3%).

Psychosocial assessment for different groups of patients

These assessments represent the point of view of the general practitioner. With the construction of different groups of patients, according to their own experience and according to the GHQ we have the point of view of the patient ("felt need") and the "normative need" at our disposal. Combination of the three will provide us with more understanding in the recognition of mental disorder by the general practitioner.

In table 4.5 patients are divided again in the three groups of chapter 3: those who felt no mental distress and scored low on the GHQ, those who experienced distress but scored low on the GHQ (they felt a need without being considered clinically potential cases of mental disorder) and those who paired a subjective experience of mental disturbance with a GHQ-score, indicating probable mental disorder. The proportion is given of each group of patients, whose reason for visit was assessed at least once during the three month registration as being not "purely somatic". Of course, only those patients are considered who visited their general practitioner during the registration period.

Table 4.5
Psychosocial assessment, for 3 groups of patients as indicated by their own experience of distress and the GHQ

Patient group:	N	Psychosocial assessment during 3- month registration	
No exp.of distress/ GHQ -	2004	654	(32.6%)
Exp. of distress/ GHQ -	692	328	(47.4%)
Exp. of distress/ GHQ +	515	343	(66.6%)

Of patients who did not experience mental distress, the diagnosis of about one third is assessed as being not entirely somatic at least once during the three month registration. This is the case for about half of those who experienced psychosocial distress without scoring positively on the GHQ. Of the GHQ-cases, the diagnosis of about two-thirds is assessed as being not entirely somatic at least once.

Within each of the three groups of patients, the relationship between patient characteristics and a psychosocial assessment by the general practitioner is investigated.

Table 4.5 summarizes the results of cross-tabulation analysis. To save room, the cross-tabulations are given at the end of the chapter[4] and only the resulting chi-squares and significance levels are given below in table 4.6. In general, diagnoses of divorced persons, women, patients of middle age, less well-educated people and incapacitated people are more frequently assessed as being not entirely somatic. However, when these relationships are considered for the three groups separately, most of them disappear for the most severe group, those who combine the experience of feelings of mental distress with a high GHQ-score. Thus, for those patients who were not indicated by themselves nor by the GHQ as suffering from mental distress, the general practitioner tends to assess complaints of women, middle aged people, divorced and incapacitated persons more easily as being not entirely somatic. Complaints of patients who *feel* distressed but who are not indicated as such by the GHQ, are more easily considered psychological when these patients are divorced, less well educated, publicly insured or incapacitated. But in the group of patients who combine experience of mental distress with an objective indication by the GHQ, psychological assessment is independent of those characteristics (with the exception of education).

Table 4.6
Patient characteristics and GP-assessment "not somatic"
for three different groups of patients.
Chi-squares and levels of significance

Patient characteristic:	No Experiences of mental distress /GHQ:- /GHQ:-	Experiences of ment. distr. GHQ:+	Experiences of ment. distr.
Sex	$X^2 = 9.17$	$X^2 = 1.64$	$X^2 = .32$
(df = 1)	($p < .01$)	(n.s.)	(n.s.)
Age	$X^2 = 18.46$	$X^2 = 5.29$	$X^2 = 5.82$
(df = 4)	($p < .001$)	(n.s.)	(n.s.)
Marital Status	$X^2 = 15.6$	$X^2 = 9.42$	$X^2 = 2.44$
(df = 3)	($p < .01$)	($p < .05$)	(n.s.)
Education	$X^2 = 10.8$	$X^2 = 14.35$	$X^2 = 13.4$
(df = 6)	(n.s.)	($p < .05$)	($p < .05$)
Insurance	$X^2 = .93$	$X^2 = 4.8$	$X^2 = 1.5$
(df = 1)	(n.s.)	($p < .05$)	(n.s.)
Employment status	$X^2 = 18.07$	$X^2 = 12.6$	$X^2 = 8.45$
(df = 6)	($p < .05$)	($p < .05$)	(n.s.)
Urbanization	$X^2 = 6.6$	$X^2 = 1.0$	$X^2 = 1.29$
(df = 3)	(n.s.)	(n.s.)	(n.s.)

Interdoctor-variation in the assessment "not purely somatic" and the recognition of GHQ-cases

In the introduction of this chapter the inter-doctor variation with regard to psychosocial assessments has been mentioned. The figures given in the last subchapters were averages, taking all registrating GPs together. These averages stand for a broad range of individual assessments. Figure 4.8 shows this range for the three indices, defined by Goldberg and Huxley and introduced at the beginning of this chapter[5].

As we explained there, bias stands for the proportion of visiting patients of an individual general practitioner whose diagnoses at least once were assessed as being not purely somatic. The median is 41% but the range goes from 12% to 84%. Some general practitioners seldom consider the problem only physical by nature, others nearly always.

On average, two thirds of all patients identified by the GHQ as probable cases of mental disorder are recognized at least once as such by the general practitioner. However, some of them only recognized one third, others "hit" the full hundred per cent. We could not establish differences in characteristics of the general practitioners related to these differences in identification index.

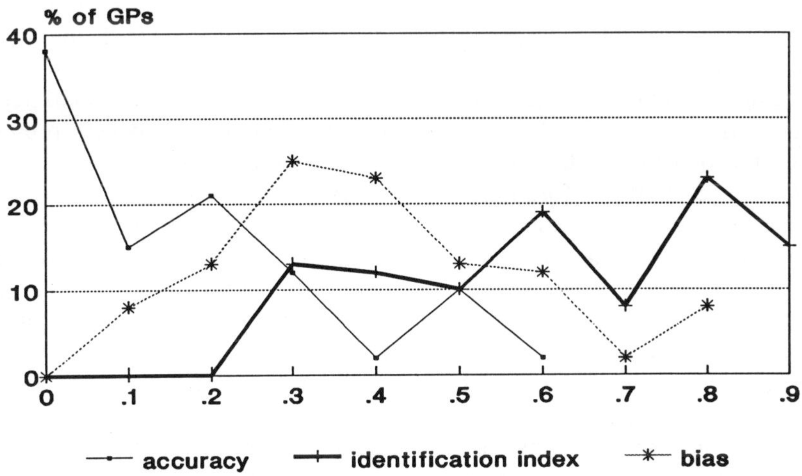

Figure 4.8 Distribution of bias, identification index and accuracy of individual GPs

Finally, the generally low correlations between general practitioner-assessment and GHQ (the median of the phi-coefficient used indicating "accuracy" is .18) demonstrates that a high identification rate generally goes together with many "false positives": patients assessed sometimes as "not purely somatic", while their GHQ is below threshold.

Recognition of mental disorder by the general practitioner

Some interesting conclusions may be drawn from the results of the last paragraphs about the ability of general practitioners to recognize the presence of mental disorder, as measured by the GHQ, or mental problems, as experienced by the patient.

As far as we can speak about sensitivity, the average general practitioner is most sensitive to the mental disorder as the GHQ indicates it. This is not surprising, as we saw already in the former chapter that these patients seem to suffer more severely than those who report feelings of mental distress but score low on the GHQ. Two-thirds of those patients who are indicated by the GHQ as probably suffering from mental disorder, insofar as they reached the doctor's office, are diagnosed at least once during three months as not entirely somatic. If we take the GHQ as the indicator of the psychopathology from a psychiatric point of view, the general practitioner seems to recognize two-thirds of the psychiatric diseases. However, these "recognized" GHQ-cases (343 in table 4.5) constitute only one quarter of all the patients whose complaints have been assessed at least once during three months as being "not entirely somatic". Complaints of one third of the patients who indicated no feelings of distress during the health interview and scored below GHQ-threshold, were nevertheless assessed at least once as being not entirely somatic. When interpreting this result, we should keep in mind that the health interview was an assessment at one moment in time, while the patient registration (and assessment by the general practitioner) lasted three months. Moreover, it is always possible that patients present themselves on one particular occasion as being tense or complaints are not easily explained by physical illness, while the patient in general does not feel mentally disturbed at all. This phenomenon also explains the low accuracy rates, reported in figure 4.8, compared with the much higher identification indices: diagnoses of many patients who were not identified by the GHQ are nevertheless sometimes assessed as not purely somatic during the three months registration.

Another substantial number of psychosocial assessments (328 or again one quarter) is given to patients who are, from a psychiatric point of view not probable cases of mental disorder, but who did in fact experience feelings of distress within the period concerned. Taking these also in account, we might conclude that about half of the patients whose complaints were assessed in a psychosocial way, were either from a psychiatric point of view or in their own view in need for mental help.

The probability of a psychosocial assessment thus increases from "no distress" via "experience of distress without being a GHQ-case" to a "GHQ-case which has the largest probability of being "detected". Another phenomenon to be discussed in this respect are the results from table 4.6. Psychosocial assessment in the former groups is more dependent on patient characteristics than in the group of GHQ-cases. The assessment of a diagnosis "not entirely somatic" relies heavily on patient characteristics such as age, sex, and working status, particularly when patients do not report feelings of distress themselves. Some stereotyping seems to be involved in these cases, as already has been remarked in the introductory section. Psychosocial assessment of GHQ-cases on the other hand is largely independent of patient characteristics, which indicates that a general practitioner is to a certain extent sensitive to the same latent stimuli as the GHQ.

Output: incidence and prevalence of diagnoses of mental disorder by general practitioners

The result of this process of problem presentation, assessment and translation is the diagnosis, made by the general practitioner. Table 4.7 gives the proportion of patients who received a diagnosis within the ICPC-chapters "Psychological" and "Social" during three months registration, divided according to reported level of distress into the three well-known categories.

In general, 17.7% of all the visitors were diagnosed at least once within one of these two chapters. 10% of those not reporting any feeling of mental distress during the interview got a psychological or social diagnosis during the three month registration. 20% of those reporting such feelings, without scoring above GHQ-threshold were diagnosed in such way, while this was also the case with more than 40% of the GHQ-cases.

The background characteristics of patients with psychological or social diagnoses in the three different groups show an even greater lack of differences, than as we observed with regard of the assessment "not purely somatic". We see in this table no differences between categories when patients are experiencing feelings of distress themselves or when the GHQ indicates a large probability of psychopathology. If such a self-reported feeling of distress did not exist, women, divorced and middle-aged people would have higher chances on a psychosocial diagnosis. In other words: where "felt need" and "normative need" in the population were strongly related to patient-characteristics, this relationship becomes weaker when we look at the demand for help and disappears largely when the general practitioner's diagnosis is considered, particularly for patients with a large probability of mental disorder.

Table 4.7
Patients with a psychological or social diagnosis, split up according to level of distress and patient-characteristics

		No distress GHQ: - (2004)	Feelings of distress GHQ: - (692)	Feeling of distress GHQ:+ (515)
Total		10.1%	20.8%	42.3%
Sex	Male	8.4%*	19.8%	47.0%
	Female	11.8%	21.3%	40.4%
Age	15-24	6.8%**	13.9%	36.7%
	25-44	10.0%	24.0%	38.8%
	45-64	13.4%	19.2%	48.6%
	65-74	6.0%	21.3%	52.9%
	75+	16.7%	25.6%	34.3%
Marital status	Married	9.5%**	22.7%	40.4%
	Divorced	25.0%	20.5%	43.9%
	Widows/widowers	9.3%	18.2%	50.8%
	Unmarried	10.4%	17.0%	41.8%
Highest level of education completed	Only primary school	9.4%	20.9%	44.3%
	Techn./Voc Training 12-16 yrs	8.8%	23.2%	45.4%
	Lower gen.sec. education	10.5%	16.7%	40.7%
	Techn./Voc.Tr. 16-18 yrs	10.1%	33.3%	41.5%
	Higher gen.sec. education	13.3%	12.8%	24.1%
	Techn./Voc Train. 18+	10.5%	14.0%	37.9%
	University	14.3%	-	25.0%
Employment status	Student/Conscript	4.3%	15.7%	30.6%
	Housewife/man	9.5%	24.1%	39.8%
	Unemployed	5.6%	25.0%	29.2%
	Incapacitated	12.7%	17.6%	42.5%
	Retired	9.7%	21.2%	46.2%
	Employed	11.4%	21.1%	42.9%
Insurance	Public	10.3%	19.0%	40.7%
	Private	10.1%	21.5%	43.0%
Urbanization	Rural	10.2%	16.8%	40.0%
	Suburban	10.2%	23.1%	42.8%
	Urban	10.1%	24.1%	41.2%
	3 Large cities	9.0%	17.8%	41.2%

** $p < .01$ * $p < .05$

We should realize of course that in this table part of the variation between patients with different characteristics has been taken away by the split-up in subgroups with different feelings of distress and GHQ-score, which groups themselves are highly correlated with the patient characteristics concerned.

It should also be kept in mind that the last tables, split up according to level of mental distress of the patient, as measured during the health interview, have patients as denominator. Each patient counts once, in contradistinction to the following morbidity analyses of the whole population, in which case the episode of illness is the denominator and some patients may be counted several times.

Incidence and prevalence of psychological and social diagnoses

To present morbidity figures in a meaningful way, comparable to the relevant literature, the following data have been derived from the complete Survey of Morbidity and Interventions in General Practice. Thus far, only the results of the morbidity registration of the interviewed sample (N = 10.787) has been used. This approach has made it possible to take into account the GHQ-scores and experience of mental distress of the patients, which were assessed during the interview. This sample, however, has its numerical limitations, when specific diagnoses are wanted.

In the following tables, we present incidences and prevalences per 1000 persons in the population at risk (= the practice population) and per 1000 persons who actually contacted their general practitioner. In order to calculate these figures, episodes of illness have been constructed, each episode counting once. Thus a patient consulting the general practitioner three times during registration with, let us say, a depressive disorder, is counted once with an episode of depressive disorder. But a patient, who is once diagnosed as "depressed", once as "relational problems" and once as "addicted", and these have been considered as three different episodes of illness, will be counted three times. Requests for prescriptions, even if the receptionist attended to them, are included, especially increasing prevalence of anxiety and sleeping disorders. All episodes which are new or are new outbreaks of existing disorders are counted as adding to the incidence. Each episode, new or existing, is counted when calculating the prevalence. See for more details chapter 2.

The three-month incidence of psychological morbidity is 24.01/1000 persons at risk and 55.25/1000 patients with a general practitioner-contact. The incidence of social problems is 7.76/1000 on population level and 15.08/1000 on contact level.

Incidence figures may be multiplied, so on population level there are 96 psychological diagnoses and 31 social problems per thousand persons in one year.

Table 4.8
Incidence and prevalence of psychological and social diagnoses, and patient characteristics (/1000 in a 3-month period)

Patient characteristics		Incidence		Prevalence	
		Population	Visitors*	Population	Visitor*
Total:		32.7	75.4	123.5	284.0
Sex	male	24.8	68.0	84.4	231.4
	female	40.0	80.2	158.8	318.7
Age	15-24	24.0	63.3	42.5	112.3
	25-44	35.7	89.2	90.4	226.0
	45-64	35.8	79.0	164.6	362.6
	65+	32.5	56.4	260.5	452.6
Marital status	Married	32.1	62.2	117.8	228.6
	Divorced	68.3	119.2	232.9	406.6
	Widows/widowers	44.1	61.4	335.6	467.4
	Unmarried	26.8	61.2	68.1	155.3
Highest level of education completed	primary	36.5	72.8	194.4	387.2
	secondary	33.0	78.6	95.5	227.3
	higher	28.9	84.0	74.3	215.7
Employment status	Student/Conscript				
	Housewife/man	41.7	85.8	150.7	310.1
	Unemployed	41.9	100.7	114.6	275.0
	Incapacitated	44.3	82.8	255.8	477.7
	Retired	31.8	56.5	251.1	446.4
	Employed	33.3	84.7	80.3	203.8
Insurance	Public	36.3	76.9	141.6	299.8
	Private	26.6	72.7	94.2	257.5
Urbanization	Rural	27.8	53.6	126.9	245.0
	Suburban	33.3	63.6	117.9	225.2
	Urban	39.5	74.2	126.1	232.9
	3 Large cities	40.3	70.6	126.1	261.0

* Persons with at least one contact during the 3-month registration

In table 4.8 diagnoses from ICPC-chapters "Psychological" and "Social" have been taken together. This table shows, at population level, a peak in psychiatric incidence for adults, for women, for divorced people, for the less well-educated, for the unemployed and housewives and for the publicly-insured. Comparison of the incidence rates with the number of visitors as numerator demonstrates that some of the differences can be attributed to differences in contact rates of some categories. For example, the difference between publicly and privately- insured persons at the population level is largely a result of the higher contact rate of the former and the difference almost disappears when only visitors are counted in the numerator. On the other hand, the already outstanding position of the 25-44 year old at population level, becomes more outstanding at contact level, due to the fact that this age group is relatively underrepresented in respect of consultation with their general practitioners.

Actually, if we are interested in general practitioner preferences in making psychiatric diagnoses for certain categories, we should look at the figures with the number of visitors as a numerator. Because, in case of the insurance example, the population-based difference between publicly and privately insured seems to be a result of different illness behaviour of the both groups. When there has been a contact, most of the difference has disappeared. On the other hand, for the sake of comparability with other studies, population based figures are to be preferred.

Table 4.9
Incidence and prevalence rates for specific diagnoses
(/1000 population in a 3-month period)

	Incidence		Prevalence	
Anxiety	4.12		27.10	
(Anxious, nervous)		(3.88)		(26.23)
(Anxiety disorder)		(.24)		(.87)
Sleeping disorder	1.00		26.80	
Depression	2.93		12.67	
(Neurotic depression)		(2.49)		(10.76)
(Depressive feeling)		(.44)		(1.91)
Overwork/Neurasthenia	4.60		7.90	
Stress	2.09		5.76	
Tension headache	2.24		3.65	
Hyperventilation syndrome	2.26		3.61	
Addictions (alcohol, drugs, tobacco, medicine)	1.09		3.51	
Illness/death partner	.50		3.23	
Relational problems	1.13		2.20	
Employment problems	.88		1.53	
Dementia	.19		1.23	
Schizophrenia	.09		.60	

Table 4.9 gives the incidence and prevalence rates for a number of specific diagnoses in general practice.

One striking feature in table 4.9 is the major role of so called "symptom diagnoses" (see also chapter 1 about diagnoses in primary care settings). general practitioners rarely make use of psychiatric nosological diagnoses, except for neurotic depression, and limit themselves in most cases to the symptom presented. So, although the prevalence of mental disorder, according to the general practitioner's diagnosis is rather high, they perceive in fact little severe psychopathology, or at least, the do not label it in such a fashion. Furthermore, it should be mentioned again in this respect that requests for (repeat-)prescriptions will have given rise to a great number of "sleeping problems" and "anxious, nervous"

Another remarkable characteristic of a number of the most popular diagnoses is the high prevalence/incidence ratio: less than a quarter of all episodes of depression, less than fifteen per cent of anxiety episodes and less than five per cent of sleeping disorders are new diagnoses. On the other hand, a number of more event-related diagnoses, such as overwork, tension headache, relational and working problems, count at least fifty per cent new episodes.

The distribution of patient characteristics over the most common diagnoses, presented in table 4.9 is presented in more detail at the end of the chapter[6]. When we take a closer examination of the background-characteristics of patients with specific diagnoses, it becomes clear that some diagnoses share the same typology of patients. Figure 4.9 presents a short summary.

For "anxious,nervous", "anxiety disorder", "depressive feelings", "neurotic depression", "sleeping disorder" and "illness/death of partner" the following typology holds true: prevalence increases with age, far more women than men are affected by it (odds > 2), there is an overrepresentation of low education, diagnoses are most prevalent among widows/widowers, followed by divorced and they are most prevalent among retired and incapacitated people.

Almost their opposite are people with "overwork/neurasthenia" and "employment problems", who are mostly adults (25 - 64), working and well-educated. The preponderance of women is less articulate, in the case of employment problems there are relatively more men. Although the diagnosis-symptom "stress" appeared related to overwork/ neurasthenia, the patients are significantly different in some respects. Patients with "stress" are in a larger majority women, they are older adults (45-64), they are relatively often incapacitated and less well-educated.

Diagnoses: *Anxious, nervous/ Anxiety disorder/ Depressive feelings/ Neurotic depression/ Sleeping disorder/ Death/illness partner*
Age: increasing with age
♂ : ♀: larger than 1:2
Education: lower level of education > second./higher education*
Working status: housewives incapac. retired > rest
Marital status: divorced, widow/widower > rest (sleeping problems: widowed > divorced)

Diagnoses:	*Overwork Neurasthenia*	*Employment problems*	*Stress*
Age:	top: 25 - 65 years	idem	idem
♂ : ♀:	♀ > ♂ (less than 2:1)	♂ > ♀	♀ > ♂ (less than 2:1)
Education:	second./higher	idem	lower educ.
Working status:	working, incapac. housewife	working incapac.	housewife incapac.
Marital status:	divorced > rest	rest > widowed	divorced > (un)married

Diagnoses: *Tension headache, hyperventilation, relational problems*
Age: < 65 years
♂ : ♀: ♀ > ♂ (less than 2:1)
Education: no difference (hyperventilation: lower/second. > higher)
Working status: housewives, incap. unemployed > retired
Marital status: divorced > married > unmarried, widows/widowers

Diagnoses: *Dementia*
Age: > 65 years
♂ : ♀: ♀ > ♂
Education: lower level of education
Working status: retired
Marital status: widows/widowers

Diagnoses: *Addiction*
Age: 25 - 65 years
♂ : ♀: ♂ = ♀
Education: no differences
Working status: incapac. unemployed > rest
Marital status: divorced > rest

Diagnoses: *Schizophrenia*
Age: increases with age
♂ : ♀: ♂ = ♀
Education: lower level of education
Working status: incapac > retired, unemployed > housewive > rest
Marital status: divorced > widows/widowers, unmarried > married

* A difference is reported, if the odds-ratio (in the figures of note 6) exceeds 1.7

Figure 4.9 The most common psychological and social diagnoses in six typologies

Patients with "tension headache", "hyperventilation" and "relational problems" share the fact that they are relatively seldom above 65 and mostly women. Divorced persons have higher probabilities than married people, who have again a higher probability than unmarried and widows/widowers. Housewives and -"house men" are most at risk, especially compared with retired persons and those with paid employment.

Three diagnoses have a typology of their own: Dementia, almost exclusively people above 65 years of age, and consequently almost exclusively retired persons and overrepresentation of the less well-educated and publicly insured. Women are also in this case overrepresented. Addiction is - besides "working problems" - the only diagnosis with a male majority. It is most predominant among adults (25-64), less well-educated and publicly insured persons. Relatively many of them are divorced. Unemployed and incapacitated persons are at a high risk compared with working people, housewives and -men, and especially retired people. The typology of the last one, "Schizophrenia" is in some respects equal to the one for affective disorders, but there are some differences. There are no sex differences in the first place. Secondly, affective disorders are predominantly found among incapacitated and retired persons, while schizophrenia is relatively often found, in addition to among incapacitated, among the unemployed. Schizophrenia is also relatively speaking most often found among the divorced. Patients with schizophrenia resemble perhaps most the addicted patients.

Conclusions

In this chapter we have considered the second and third level of the Goldberg and Huxley model. This is a critical stage in the translation of need (be it the "felt need" of the patient or the "normative need" assessed by the professional) into a demand for help. Our analyses clarified some issues concerning the actual demands, put forward by patients and the added value of the diagnostic process of the general practitioner. Before considering this matters in greater detail, we shall first compare our results with those of previous research.

Previous research

17.7% of those of the interviewed sample who contacted their general practitioner was diagnosed at least once as psychological or social. This figure should be compared with figures given in table 4.4. It falls between the extremes. The prevalence rate of 284/1000 visitors with a psychological or social diagnosis, based on the entire study population is higher, first, because it has episodes of illness in the numerator instead of patients (so, one patient may count twice), second, because all requests for repeat prescriptions are taken into account, which has not been done in the interview sample. This prevalence rate sounds extremely high, but has been repeated by several other studies.

It is rather common to find a predominance of women with diagnoses of mental disorder in the literature. In fact, this finding has been repeated, but our division into three groups of patients, with or without subjective and objective levels of distress, enables us to throw an interesting light on this matter. In fact it appeared that within the majority of patients without an objective indication of mental disorder, women are more frequently diagnosed as being mentally ill, while in the GHQ+group men and women were equally diagnosed as being mentally ill.

Recalculating the "GHQ-prevalence" among doctor's visitors, 178 out of 1000 visitors appear to be GHQ-cases. This is extremely low, compared with the data from other studies, presented in table 4.1. Each visitor only counted once; if we distribute the GHQ-scores over the contacts, allowing some patients to count once and some to count a dozen times, then the proportion of "GHQ-contacts" raises up till 225/1000 contacts. This still remains below the lowest score from previous research. A possible explanation will be the distance in time between GHQ-assessment and contact with the general practitioner. The health interviews took place in the second registration month, so theoretically this distance may be six weeks, where the GHQ should cover a distance of four weeks. However, excluding the extremes in time, allowing only for contacts within three weeks from the interview, did not change our results (Verhaak, in press). It is plausible that completing the GHQ at the very moment of help-seeking, may result in more "positive" cases than any moment earlier or later.

The assessments made by the general practitioner on the 5-point-scale, resulting in more than 30% of all diagnoses being not entirely somatic, fit within the range of six previous studies, using comparable scales. The frequent occurrence of psychosocial assessments within ICPC-chapters "General", "Digestive" and "Neurological" has been found also by van der Meer (1994) in a Dutch study among 25 general practitioners.

At last the prevalence and incidence of a number of ICPC-diagnoses, obtained from the complete database of the National Survey, need some comments.

To compare our figures, collected during three months, with other surveys that present incidence- and prevalence rates on a yearly basis, we can multiply our incidence figures by four to get the 1-year incidence. As this is not possible with prevalence figures, we shall concentrate on the incidence figures. Multiplying our over-all 3-month incidence of 32.7/1000 gives us an incidence of 130.8/1000. This is somewhat higher than Lamberts (1991), based on 20 Dutch Academic practices, who reports 10%, and the third English National Study with 7%. However, the last figures are from 1981-1982. It is more in line with another Dutch academic practice network in Nijmegen with 12% incidence among men and 16% among women (van de Lisdonk et al. 1990).

Our specific figures about anxious/nervous and anxiety disorders (16.5) and depression (11.9) appear in line with Lamberts (16 resp. 10) and the English National Study (19.3 resp. 16.9). The 1-year incidence for stress is 8.4, whereas Lamberts and the English National Study report 9. Addiction figures are comparable as well.

Discussion

As we observed already in the previous chapter, a substantial part of those who feel distressed (according to themselves) or who are distressed (according to the objective screening-instrument, GHQ) arrive at the general practitioner's office within a few months. We also noticed that the probabilities of such an arrival are highest for those who combine a subjective feeling of distress during the last weeks with an elevated score on the GHQ. However, only a minority of those who indicated mental distress and visited their general practitioner, explicitly brought forward psychological of social reasons for their visit. And again, the probability of doing such was highest for those who combined a felt need and a normative need, subjective feelings and objective indicators.

Furthermore, it was striking to find that a number of categories, which proved to be at a higher risk for mental distress, were not relatively more inclined to present psycho-social reasons for visit. Thus, women, widows/widowers, incapacitated or unemployed and publicly insured persons appear to have equal chances to express psychosocial complaints as men, married persons, persons in paid employment or privately-insured persons, although in general the former categories appear at greater risks for mental disorder.

In analyzing the process of decision making by the general practitioner, we discovered that there is certainly no one-to-one relationship between complaints, expressed by the patient, and diagnoses given by the general practitioner. Complaints about the digestive system, in particular, such as stomach-pain and gastritis and general complaints such as fatigue and general feelings of ill health end relatively often with a psychological diagnosis by the general practitioner. It is gratifying that such "switches" occurred especially among patients who were indicated by the GHQ as possible cases of mental disorder. The psychosocial connotation of these kinds of symptoms can also be concluded from the fact that nearly half of the diagnoses within the ICPC-chapters "General" and "Digestive" have been assessed on a 5-point scale as "not entirely physical".

This general practitioner-assessment provides the general practitioner with another means of expressing his judgment that the symptoms presented actually indicate psychological distress. Again, this judgment was most frequently given for patients who combined feelings of distress and a high GHQ, followed by patients who felt distressed without crossing the GHQ-threshold.

Here we find lack of relationship between patient-characteristics and general practitioner's judgement. Although in the previous chapter marital status, sex and employment status significantly influenced the probability of being a GHQ-case, the chances that a GHQ-case will be assessed by the general practitioner as having a not-strictly somatic illness are independent of the subjects being a man or a woman, a housewife or being in paid employment. Strangely enough, those relationships can be observed when the patient is not suffering psychological distress, according to his own information or the GHQ. As was mentioned earlier, when apparently the cues of psychological distress are lacking, a general practitioner has the tendency to stereotype women and older people.

The same kind of phenomenon can be observed when we take the relationship between patient-characteristics and a psychological or social diagnosis into account. Within the group who did not have any mental distress, women, elderly and divorced persons had a higher probability of such a diagnosis than their opposites. Within the groups who in fact had any indication of distress, these relationships are lacking.

The majority of diagnoses given fall into the domain of so called "symptom diagnoses", anxious/nervous, sleeping disturbances and feelings of stress being the most important. Together with neurotic depression these diagnoses are typically given to older women relatively often with a low level of education. In case of younger women, tension headache, hyperventilation and relational problems are probable diagnoses. Overwork/neurasthenia and problems related to work on the other hand, are diagnosed where adult working males with relatively often a higher education are dominant. In absolute figures, many of these symptom diagnoses are given to patients who did not report feelings of distress rather recently, but nevertheless presented symptoms to their general practitioner. As many of these symptoms can point to more than one "official" diagnosis within the DSM-III domain, we have got a picture of a "lucky bag", filled with symptoms, a "saucerful of secrets", from which each diagnostician can draw at his own discretion.

This impression is strengthened by other evidence. In a recent Dutch study, Terluin (1994) made an inventory of symptoms experienced by patients diagnosed by their general practitioner as "overwork", "somatization", "anxiety", "depressed" and "mildly psychosocial" respectively. He was able to cluster their symptoms into two categories: a-specific distress (including symptoms like fatigue, hypersomnia, insomnia, demoralization, and feeling tense) and neurotic symptoms: depressive feelings, manifestations of anxiety and somatization. Neurotic symptoms were always accompanied by distress symptoms but not vice versa. Patients diagnosed as "mildly psychosocial" had moderate distress and low neurotic symptoms. Patients who were diagnosed as "overworked" had high distress and relatively low neurotic symptoms. Patients with diagnoses such as "depression", "anxiety", and "somatization" had high distress combined with high neurotic symptoms.

General distress is far more abundant in general practice than specific neurotic disorders, but its components are the ones that constitute DSM-III diagnoses. Furthermore, we are confronted with the same hierarchy as that introduced in the first chapter, discussing Foulds and Hodiamont: severe mental disorder is always combined with less severe, a-specific symptoms. Such circumstances will easily lead to overestimation of severe mental disorder, when we have to rely on mere symptom-counting.

Or, in other words, the symptoms for DSM-III diagnoses are available in general practice settings, but they should be interpreted in their right context. Presumably GPs often consider this context not so alarming as to label the patients with "real" psychiatric diagnoses.

Epilogue

The following research questions have been answered in this chapter: What demands for help result from felt and normative needs and to what extent are these needs recognized as such by general practitioners. Let us first consider the conditions that promote the chances of demanding help and recognition. Secondly we will discuss the reasons for not demanding help or recognizing a need, which is assumed to be present by psychiatric standards.

What is becoming more and more clear is that the pathway to a psychological or social diagnosis is most accessible to those who are in need according the professional psychiatric standard. They have the highest probability of consulting the general practitioner, they have the highest probability, if they do consult him, of reporting psychosocial complaints, and accordingly, they have the highest probability of a psychological of social diagnosis. The chances for people who report feelings of distress without being identified by the GHQ, are in all respects smaller. Furthermore, assessment of their symptoms as psychiatric rests partly on stereotyping by the general practitioner. The chances for people without feelings of distress are, again, substantially smaller. But, as the latter group is numerically by far the largest, many people without distress are presenting psychological symptoms and are diagnosed accordingly. Perhaps it is common for many elderly women to have sleep disturbances or feelings of nervousness and to discuss them with their general practitioner, without labelling themselves as "feeling distressed". On the other hand, what should be added to this conclusion is that the majority of those in the population who are in need, according those professional standards, are not diagnosed as being mentally disturbed at all, and this is mainly due to the fact that they either do not seek any help at all, or do not put forward a psychological demand for help.

This chapter made clear that there are several ways to reach a psychological or social diagnosis. A psychosocial diagnosis may originatc from psychosocial complaints, but it is not unusual that complaint of a more physical nature are evaluated by the general practitioner as essentially psychological or social too. Furthermore, a considerable proportion of diagnoses with the ICPC-chapters "General", "Digestive" and "Neurology" is assigned a psychosocial meaning as well.

With all these additions to the original demand for help, we cannot maintain that it's a patient's world. The psychiatric point of view appears to gain the upper hand, as the general practitioner is especially inclined to add psychological assessments and diagnoses to patients who should be in psychiatric need according to the GHQ. The next chapter will reveal the consequences this may have for the management of the problems detected.

At last some comments should be made about the result that many patients, indicated by the GHQ as possible cases of mental disorder, do not make demands for help, nor are they diagnosed as mentally disturbed by the general practitioner. A-specific distress has been mentioned as an experience many patients have, that does not necessarily have to lead to a psychological diagnosis, though it may very well lead, temporarily, to a high GHQ-score or even a DSM-III diagnosis (assuming the symptoms are manifold enough). During a clinical interview it will become clear that no action is needed - a conclusion the general practitioner might have reached during his interview too - and the patient is counted among the false positives.

Accordingly, two tendencies have become clear in this chapter. People who are more in need (in their own view and that of the GHQ) have a higher chance of demanding psychosocial help from their general practitioner and have also higher chance of being diagnosed as having a psychological or social problem.

On the other hand, many people may have a-specific distress symptoms, resulting in a high GHQ-score, but do not constitute a case of mental illness in a clinical sense. Partly they have the same symptoms, patients with a "real" depression or anxiety disorder have, but they may miss the essential thing, and therefore, they may not need the treatment a truly depressed patient requires. And after all, the possibility of treatment is the purpose a diagnosis has been made for.

Notes

1. The following abbreviations have been used for the several existing interview schedules resp. classification schemes:
   CIS: Clinical Interview Schedule
   PSE: Present State Examination
   DSM-III; Diagnostic Statistical Manual, third version
   SADS-L: Schizofrenic and Affective disorder Schedule (Lifetime version)
   DIS: Diagnostic Interview Schedule.

2. For morc information on this survey, see chapter 3.

3. Categories are from Goldberg and Bridges, 1987. The older version also contained remainder categories like "miscellaneous" and "parent with sick child". These have been omitted. The old categories "physical illness in a neurotic personality" and "physical illness with associated psychiatric disturbance" are apparently taken together in category 2. In Verhaak's study, the middle categories are not comparable.

4. **Table 4.10**

Percentage of patients, whose complaints have been assessed "not somatic", split up by "feelings of distress/GHQ" and by background characteristics

		No distress	Feelings of distress	
		GHQ: -	GHQ: -	GHQ:+
Total		32.6%	47.4%	66.6%
Characteristics				
Sex	Male	29.4%**	44.1%	68.5%
	Female	35.8%	49.2%	65.8%
Age	15-24	26.0%***	38.9%	60.8%
	25-44	33.0%	48.4%	63.6%
	45-64	36.2%	51.5%	73.6%
	65-74	29.1%	43.8%	70.6%
	75+	45.6%	51.3%	62.9%
Marital status	Married	33.2%**	49.9%*	64.5%
	Divorced	51.9%	59.1%	70.7%
	Widow/widower	38.3%	47.0%	73.8%
	Unmarried	28.0%	37.7%	66.4%
Highest level of education completed	Only primary school	34.4%	46.2%*	67.6%*
	Techn./Voc Tr. 12-16yrs	31.1%	54.2%	70.0%
	Lower gen. second. educ.	38.2%	52.1%	67.8%
	Techn./Voc. Tr. 16-18yrs	30.6%	50.0%	61.0%
	Higher gen. second. educ.	31.4%	33.3%	44.8%
	Techn./Voc Training 18+	25.9%	34.0%	69.0%
	University	22.9%	-	25.0%
Employment status	Student/Conscript	22.2%*	39.2%*	52.8%
	Housewife/man	35.8%	58.2%	63.3%
	Unemployed	36.1%	60.7%	66.7%
	Incapacitated	49.1%	50.0%	82.5%
	Retired	33.9%	45.3%	66.7%
	Employed	32.3%	43.9%	68.7%
Insurance	Public	33.3%	50.1%	40.7%
	Private	31.1%	40.7%	43.0%
Urbanization	Rural	35.2%	48.7%	40.0%
	Suburban	29.5%	45.1%	42.8%
	Urban	33.6%	49.6%	41.2%
	3 Large cities	35.9%	46.7%	41.2%

*** $p < .001$ ** $p < .01$ * $p < .05$

5. In order to calculate for each GP his bias, identification index and accuracy, only the data of those GPs who had at least 20 visiting patients and 5 patients who scored above GHQ-threshold, were used.

For each patient who completed the GHQ and visited the GP in the three-month period it is possible to check whether the diagnosis of that patient was considered "not purely somatic". We get the following cross-tabulation for each GP, allowing us to compute the following indices:

		GP: "not purely somatic"	
		-	+
GHQ:	+	a	b
	-	c	d

Identification index: Proportion of GHQ-cases, assessed at least once by the GP as presenting complaints which are not purely somatic: b/(a+b). This is an approximation without making a correction for the GHQ's sensitivity. On the other hand, this correction would have been equal for all GPs

Accuracy: The correlation between GHQ and GP's assessment, expressed by the coefficient phi

Bias: The proportion of patients, assessed as being not purely somatic, as related to the total number of patients: (b+d)/(a+b+c+d).

6. **Prevalences (per 1000 population in a 3-month period)**

		anxiety	depres-sion	demen-tia	schizo-frenia	addic-tion	sleeping dis.	Tension head.	Hyper-venti-lation	relatio-nal prob	working prob	ill partner	stress	sur-menage
Total		27,09	12,67	1,23	0,60	3,51	26,80	3,65	3,61	2,20	1,53	3,23	5,46	7,90
Age	15-24	5,34	3,02	0,00	0,18	1,35	1,46	3,77	3,30	0,95	1,26	0,26	2,88	5,79
	25-44	16,89	9,64	0,01	0,59	4,55	7,21	4,24	4,62	2,89	1,91	1,90	5,48	10,00
	45-64	44,13	18,77	0,12	0,70	4,59	36,02	3,66	3,04	2,60	2,10	5,36	7,19	8,72
	65+	57,91	24,58	8,03	1,10	2,07	100,12	1,92	2,29	1,50	0,00	10,67	6,28	4,01
Sex	Male	17,23	7,66	0,85	0,55	4,22	16,26	2,35	2,53	1,48	1,97	2,33	3,86	6,78
	Female	36,04	17,20	1,58	0,65	2,89	36,34	4,83	4,60	2,85	1,14	4,93	6,90	8,93
Insurance	Public	32,40	14,43	1,23	0,75	4,23	31,55	4,29	4,07	2,27	1,69	3,83	6,13	8,37
	Private	19,24	10,27	0,97	0,32	2,17	19,67	2,68	2,64	2,01	1,41	3,23	4,32	7,62
Education	Lower	46,79	21,35	2,56	0,82	3,87	55,69	4,09	3,87	2,46	1,11	6,57	6,67	6,05
	Secondary	19,34	9,87	0,34	0,42	3,23	14,41	3,91	3,69	2,18	1,75	2,46	5,34	9,14
	Higher	11,52	6,29	0,53	0,49	2,62	11,88	2,04	2,84	1,86	2,57	1,99	4,25	9,93
Employment status	Child	3,85	1,82	0,00	0,04	0,73	1,53	2,76	2,25	0,25	0,58	0,04	1,42	2,94
	Military	0,00	2,28	0,00	0,00	0,00	0,00	1,14	0,00	1,14	1,14	0,00	1,14	2,28
	Housewive	40,34	18,33	0,03	0,63	3,11	25,13	5,72	4,72	3,61	0,45	3,80	6,99	7,86
	Unemployed	23,98	9,42	0,00	1,43	11,99	9,99	4,57	4,42	3,00	1,14	1,86	6,14	5,85
	Incapacitated	59,84	31,58	0,12	3,19	12,04	54,56	4,42	5,16	3,81	1,35	3,44	10,94	9,71
	Retired	56,82	23,93	7,27	1,06	2,18	94,89	1,87	2,32	1,49	0,07	10,42	6,17	3,92
	Paid job	14,02	8,26	0,02	0,28	3,44	7,68	3,74	3,86	2,18	2,96	1,23	5,16	11,31
Marital status	Never married	10,62	6,34	0,24	0,71	3,04	8,97	3,39	3,21	0,87	1,78	0,28	3,43	6,36
	Married	28,49	12,85	0,64	0,29	2,90	23,75	3,77	3,57	2,65	1,62	2,62	5,64	8,66
	Divorced	50,27	29,25	0,38	2,28	14,05	35,07	5,70	7,85	6,71	1,77	1,01	11,27	14,94
	Widowed	74,63	31,98	8,48	1,04	2,72	123,63	2,91	3,17	0,97	0,19	21,10	8,61	5,31
Urbanization	Rural	27,67	14,84	1,28	0,59	3,23	31,98	3,15	2,84	1,88	1,39	3,02	5,76	6,47
	Suburban	28,40	11,78	1,17	0,48	2,97	24,23	4,10	3,94	2,26	1,48	3,17	4,11	8,06
	Urban	24,56	10,24	1,46	0,78	4,41	22,57	3,86	4,08	2,31	1,84	3,30	6,34	10,71
	3 large cities	18,64	9,95	0,49	1,05	6,38	19,06	3,01	4,97	3,50	1,68	4,76	10,02	7,57

5 Treatment of mental disturbances in general practice

Introduction

When need has resulted in a demand for help and the general practitioner has diagnosed the reason for help-seeking as being a mental disorder, treatment by the general practitioner is responsible for the next steps in the help-seeking process. The general practitioner may discuss his psychosocial assumptions with the patient and choose between treatment by himself or a referral. If the general practitioner decides to refer to specialized mental health care, the patient will enter the fourth level of Goldberg and Huxley's pathway to mental health care, considering him- or herself as a "case of mental illness". If, at the other hand, the general practitioner does not make his conjectures about the psychosocial character of vague somatic complaints explicit, the patient will continue to evaluate his condition in physical terms.

When a general practitioner has arrived at the conclusion that a diagnosis of "mental disorder" is justified or at least that psychosocial aspects play an important role, treatment can been categorized in the following ways:
Talking to the patient:
- "therapeutic listening", counselling
- short-term "psychotherapy", focused on specific problem and behaviour change
- patient education
- advice

Medication:
- anti-depressants
- anxiolytics and hypnotics
- other psychotropic drugs
- other medication

Referral:
- mental health (psychiatry, regional institutes for mental health, private

psychologists)
- social work.

A review of literature

Orleans et al. (1985) asked 350 American family doctors in a questionnaire about the prevalence and treatment of psychiatric disorders. Physicians reported treating most problems themselves, usually through a combination of psychotropic drugs, advice and reassurance. Very frequently, they report treating their mentally disturbed patients with advice, reassurance or supportive problem solving. Fairly often they prescribe anti-depressants and anxiolytics. The majority never or rarely makes appointments for two or more extended interviews. A referral is considered in no more than 10 - 25 per cent of the affected patients, mostly to psychiatrists and mental health centres.

The three most commonly cited obstacles to providing psychiatric treatment are patients' resistance to referral to a mental health specialist and to a diagnosis of mental disorder, together with a lack of time from the side of the family practice physician.

Jencks (1985) analyzed data from the American National Ambulatory Medical Care Survey, a registration during one week of office-based primary care contacts, containing 40,000 contacts. In 3.3% of these contacts the reason for visit was mental health, in 5.6% there was a mental disorder diagnosis, in 6.8% psychotropic drugs are being prescribed and in 3.2% psychotherapy was recorded. A remarkable result is half of the prescriptions of psychotropic drugs are prescribed without a mental health reason for the visit or a formal mental disorder diagnosis. In the same way, about half of the psychotherapy was given when there was no mental health reason for the visit or diagnosis. Visits in which any combination of mental health treatments was provided without diagnosis were more likely to be for non-acute problems and for older patients.

Schurman et al. (1985) also used NAMC-data to describe treatment of mental illness by non-psychiatrists (mostly primary care physicians). Diagnostic services during a so called mental illness visit included a lot of physical examination but a mental status examination in only 6.4% of the consultations. Therapeutic services include drugs in 77.7% of the cases, medical counselling in 33.9%, psychotherapy - therapeutic listening in 24.8% and social counselling in 12.4%. All these services, except psychotherapy, were performed for the most part by non-psychiatrists, confronting a psychiatric diagnosis, rather than by psychiatrists.

In the Groningen "eerstelijnsproject" [primary care project] (Ormel et al. 1990, 1991) treatment by the general practitioner of 73 recognized cases (PSE) and 33 non-recognized cases was recorded. Of the former, 47%

received psychotropic drugs, 23% received counselling and 22% were referred to a mental health agency. A further 23% were referred to a medical specialist. Of the latter, 21% received psychotropic drugs and 6% counselling (compare Jenck's results above). 21% were referred to a medical specialist.

For 241 patients with new psychosocial problems Van der Meer (1994) reported prescription of tranquilizers in 13%, anti-depressants in 5% and hypnotics in 3% of the cases. A referral was recorded in 3% to social work and in another 3% to RIAGG or a psychiatrist.

In our own research (Verhaak 1986, Verhaak and Wennink 1990), we made a distinction between patients with a psychosocial diagnosis and patients with a somatic diagnosis, considered not as purely somatic by the general practitioner. 90% of the cases in the former category received some kind of psychosocial treatment from the general practitioner. However, in only 60% of the cases with physical diagnoses considered not purely somatic by the general practitioner is this psychosocial assessment visible in the treatment. In the remaining cases the general practitioners did not reveal their suspicions in their actions and limited themselves to the somatic aspects of the complaint. When psychosocial aspects were treated, in 8% of the cases, it was by prescription for psychotropic drugs and in 1% of the cases by referral to a mental health agency. In most cases the response of the general practitioner consisted in talking to the patient. In 30% of the cases in a passive way (listening, reassuring, counselling), in 20% in a more active way (exploring, short term "psychotherapy"). The less prominent role of psycho-tropic drugs in this last study, compared to the American studies discussed earlier, is mainly due to the broader definition of "mental illness", when compared with definition in the former studies.

In summary, primary care physicians in general rely heavily on their own efforts, consisting primarily of counselling and prescribing drugs, rather than a referral. In the following we shall consider the treatment given to patients with a psychological or social diagnosis and the possible differences in this respect between several categories of patient.

Management of psychological and social diagnoses

To get a major overview, we start with the data from the complete Survey of Morbidity and Interventions. Within the three months of registration of patients with a psychological or social diagnosis, the following treatment was recorded (table 5.1).

In both cases (psychological and social diagnoses) a lot of talking is involved. About one third of the psychological diagnoses and slightly more than ten per cent of the social diagnoses were treated with psychotropic drugs. A mental health referral can be observed in four per cent of the cases. We may conclude that treatment is not very specific and consists merely in listening and exploring, information giving and, in case of psychological diagnoses, drug-treatment.

Table 5.1
Treatment of patients with a psychological or a social diagnosis

	Psychological diagnosis	Social diagnosis
Therapeutic conversation		
No treatment recorded	17%	12%
Reassuring	20%	9%
Counselling (passive: therapeutic listening)	38%	57%
Counselling (active: exploring)	39%	47%
Information (on diagnosis)	24%	13%
Information (on therapy)	21%	10%
Health education	5%	4%
Advice (stopping, restarting work)	5%	4%
Medication		
No medication	60%	87%
Psychotropic drugs	35%	11%
- anxiolytics/hypnotics	25%	9%
- antidepressants	7%	1%
- other	3%	1%
Other medication	12%	4%
Referral/consultation		
Medical specialist	1.6%	.7%
Mental Health	3.7%	4.4%
- psychiatrist	1.2%	.3%
- mental health centre	1.3%	1.5%
- psychologist	0.4%	.3%
- social worker	0.8%	2.2%

In chapter 4, it was demonstrated that part of the psychological and social diagnoses were preceded by complaints that were not psychosocial but came from somatic ICPC-chapters, especially those headed "General", "Digestive", and "Neurological". In these cases the original request by the patient, leading to a psychosocial diagnosis, is not psychosocial. And this appears to have consequences for the treatment[1]. In case of psychological or social diagnoses, preceded by the patient's psychological or social complaints, more counselling (especially active) and considerably more medication and referral could be observed. In fact, about three times as many anxiolytics and hypnotics and nine times more anti-depressants were prescribed. The referral rate was nearly three times higher for patients whose psychosocial diagnosis was associated with psychosocial complaints.

Differences between patients

Treatment depends on the age of the patient, as is shown in table 5.2, where psychological and social diagnoses have been taken together. As patients get older, the frequency of "no treatment" increases, as does the frequency of passive counselling. The other categories of therapeutic conversation decrease with age, as does the proportion mental health referrals. Prescription of anxiolytics/hypnotics, on the other hand, increases, while antidepressants are increasing up to 65 years.

Table 5.2
Treatment of patients with a psychological or social diagnosis according to their age

	15-24	25-44	45-64	65-74	75+
Therapeutic conversation					
No treatment recorded	13%	13%	16%	21%	24%
Reassuring	21%	18%	17%	17%	16%
Counselling (passive: ther. listening)	37%	41%	44%	46%	43%
Counselling (active: exploring)	45%	47%	40%	35%	28%
Information (on diagnosis)	29%	23%	21%	16%	14%
Information (on therapy)	21%	20%	19%	15%	14%
Health education	5%	5%	5%	3%	3%
Advice (stopping, restarting work)	8%	7%	5%	0%	0%
Medication					
No medication	72%	67%	62%	62%	68%
Psychotropic drugs					
- anxiolytics/hypnotics	13%	19%	25%	27%	24%
- antidepressants	3%	5%	8%	7%	5%
- other	3%	3%	3%	2%	1%
Mental health referral	6%	6%	3%	1%	1%

There is hardly any difference in treatment between men and women, nor between publicly and privately-insured people. With respect to other patient characteristics, which have received our attention throughout this book, there are some relationships, but they are interpretable as a reflection of the age effect. Unmarried people (mostly younger people) receive more active counselling, fewer prescriptions and a relatively large number of them are referred. Widows/widowers (presumably older) receive more passive counselling, more medication and little referral. The same relationships as were found with age can be seen with education level, older people being less well educated than younger ones.

Interdoctorvariation in the treatment of patients with psychological or a social diagnosis

Figure 5.1 shows the differences between the 161 participating general practitioners in their application of several kinds of therapy.

The boxes in this figure represent the range between the 25th and 75th percentile. Within the box, the horizontal line represents the median. Both ends of the vertical line represent the 10th and 90th percentile respectively.

Accordingly, 10% of the participating general practitioners used counselling (active and passive) in less than 46% of the psychosocial diagnoses they made, and another 10% did this in more than 87% of the cases. The median is 67.5, consequently, half of the general practitioners counselled in more than two thirds of the cases and half of the general practitioners in less than two thirds.

Figure 5.1 shows that individual differences are large in the case of counselling and information giving, they are modest for prescription (any medicine or psychotropic drugs) and they are small for referrals. Indeed, they are so small that they required a scale multiplied by ten.

In some respects, practice characteristics are related to the general practitioner's approach to patients with a psychological or social diagnosis. Doctors working in practices with a relatively large proportion foreigners on the list have lower figures for counselling and information giving. Doctors with longer consultations (on an average) do more counselling; refer more and have lower prescription figures. Those who consider psychological treatment a typical task for the general practitioner, do more counselling and give more information. Doctors with a "democratic attitude", who consider it important to negotiate with the patients on equal terms instead as from an expert point of view do more counselling and prescribe less than their colleagues with a less "democratic attitude".

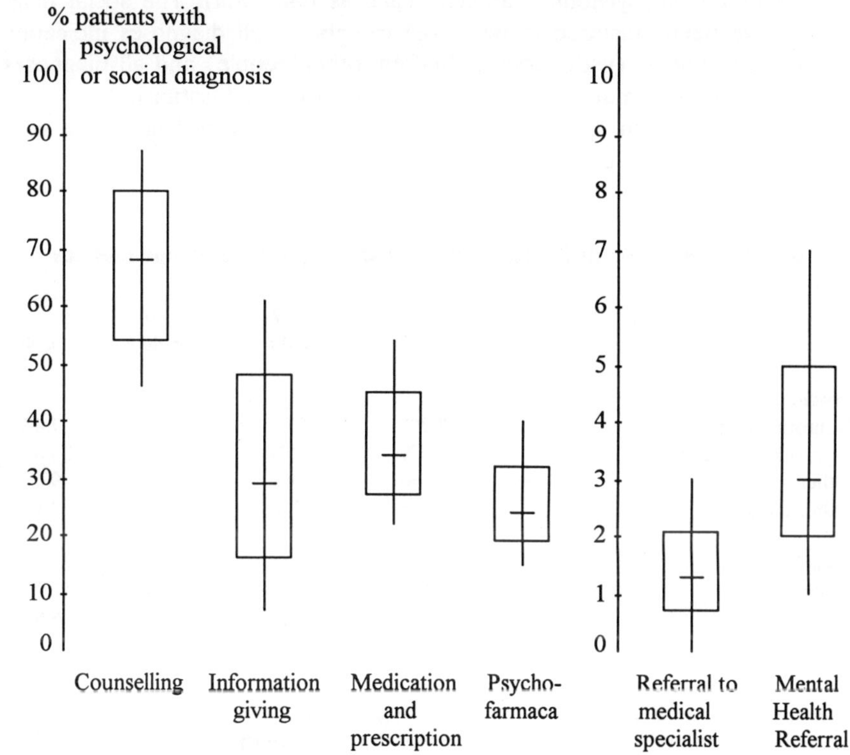

Figure 5.1 **Interdoctorvariation in treatment of patient with psychological or social diagnosis**

Referral

Although mental health referral is rare in primary care, its impact is important, as it constitutes the filter between general practice and specialist mental health care. In consequence, some extra attention will be paid to this aspect of the management of mental disorder. The relationship between referral on the one hand, and diagnosis and patient characteristics on the other can be seen in table 5.3 (cf Verhaak 1993).

In order to get a meaningful clustering of diagnoses, all neurotic mood disorders have been taken together (including anxiety, depression and stress as the most important), the much less common diagnoses indicating a psychotic disorder, such as schizophrenia and manic-depressive disorder constitute a cluster, the remaining psychological symptoms (such as tension headache and sleeping disturbances) and the remaining diagnostic categories of a non-psychotic character (such as dementia). The social diagnoses have been clustered in two large categories: all diagnoses indicating relational problems (with spouse, children, other people) and all diagnoses indicating social or material problems (finance, work, education).

Patients have been split up according to sex, and according to age with forty years as cut-off point.

Table 5.3
Referral rates for different kinds of disorder, according age and sex

	♀ ≥ 40	♀ < 40	♂ ≥ 40	♂ < 40
Psychological				
Neurotic disorders	3.7%	7.5%	5.1%	7.4%
Psychotic disorders	11.4%	15.7%	16.7%	34.0%
Other symptoms	1.4%	5.5%	2.7%	9.6%
Other diagnoses	9.7%	17.1%	8.4%	22.1%
Social				
Relational	3.5%	13.2%	6.4%	12.9%
Social/Material	3.9%	7.3%	2.2%	5.6%

Table 5.3 shows that in each age/sex category psychotic disorders and other classical psychiatric diagnostic categories had the highest referral rate. We must point out again, that these constitute about five per cent of all psychological and social diagnoses. For each diagnostic category and in both age groups, men have higher referral rates than women. And at last, for each diagnostic category and for both sexes, younger patients have higher rates than the elderly.

To complete the picture of Goldberg and Huxley's third filter, tables 5.4 and 5.5 demonstrate how referrals of different disorders and different patients are distributed over four possible mental health destinations:

Referrals with different diagnoses were not equally distributed over the four referral options. Psychiatry (psychiatric policlinics in hospitals and psychiatric hospitals as well as private psychiatrists) received the majority of the patients with "real" diagnoses, especially those with a psychotic character. Ambulatory mental health care plays an important role in these cases as well, while social work must not be neglected in case of neurotic disorders. Social work is the most important referral agency in case of relational and social/material problems, though ambulatory mental health care is almost as important in case of relational problems.

Table 5.4
Destination of referral by diagnosis

	Psychological				Social	
	Neuro tic	Psycho tic	other Sympt.	other Diagn.	Relat. probl.	Mater. probl.
Psychiatry	38%	68%	39%	42%	9%	16%
Ambulatory Mental health	29%	30%	41%	31%	39%	20%
Psychologist	11%	2%	7%	10%	7%	8%
Social work	22%	-	13%	17%	44%	56%

However, differences are not as pronounced as one might expect. The most outspoken role seems reserved for psychiatry in case of psychotic disorder. The prevalence of these diagnoses in primary care is low, so, in most decisions about a referral a general practitioner has to make, he has not such a clear choice available.

Table 5.5 shows the age-sex distribution for the four referral options. Again, the distribution contradicts the assumption of independence of age, sex and option for referral. Controlling for diagnosis does not alter this situation. Older patients were referred to psychiatry more often than younger patients. Younger men were overrepresented within ambulatory mental health care and a relatively large proportion of younger women were referred to a social worker.

Table 5.5
Destination of referral by age and sex

	♀ ≥ 40	♀ < 40	♂ ≥40	♂ <40
Psychiatry	38%	29%	45%	22%
Ambulatory	28%	31%	30%	42%
Mental Health Psychologist	8%	10%	6%	10%
Social Work	26%	31%	18%	21%

Treatment of patients with different felt and normative needs

Our interview sample provides us with the opportunity to compare the treatments, given to patients who reported experiences of mental distress during the past weeks, whether or not combined with an elevated GHQ-score. We remember from chapter 4 that the probability of a psychological or social diagnosis increased considerably if mental distress had been reported during the recent past, and again if the score was above GHQ-threshold.

Given a psychological or social diagnosis, however, the three groups do not differ that much in treatment given. Although there are slight tendencies for more counselling and medication as the subjective and objective needs increase, these differences are too small to reach any level of significance.

Table 5.6 shows the treatment given to the three groups.

Table 5.6
Treatment of patients with a psychological and social diagnosis for three categories with different degrees of mental distress

	No distress GHQ: - (N=203)	Feelings of distress GHQ: - (N=157)	Feelings of distress GHQ:+ (N=318)
Therapeutic conversation			
No treatment recorded	11%	17%	17%
Reassuring	22%	18%	19%
Counselling (passive: ther. listening)	36%	42%	43%
Counselling (active: exploring)	42%	42%	48%
Information (on diagnosis)	31%	27%	17%
Information (on therapy)	17%	20%	17%
Health education	3%	8%	2%
Advice (stopping, restarting work)	10%	5%	10%
Medication			
No medication	73%	61%	70%
Psychotropic drugs			
- anxiolytics/hypnotics	15%	23%	20%
- antidepressants	2%	6%	7%
- other	3%	3%	2%
Mental health referral	3%	3%	4%

A last point of concern is the treatment, given to patients with another than a psychological or social diagnosis. As we saw in chapter 4, in such cases the assessment by the general practitioner may be "purely somatic" or "not purely somatic". Table 5.7 shows treatment by the general practitioner in both cases.

Treatment of physical diagnoses considered partly psychosocial, differs from treatment of psycho-social diagnoses in a number of ways. The general practitioner is considerably more reluctant with counselling, passive as well as active, although there is more counselling than in the case of a physical diagnosis with a purely somatic assessment. Psychotropic drugs are rarely prescribed and a referral to a mental health agency is almost out of question. In other words, the treatment of the general practitioner gives very little inkling of his psychosocial suspicions regarding the diagnosis.

Table 5.7
Treatment of patients with a physical diagnosis, assessed as "purely somatic" or "not-purely somatic"

	Assessment "purely somatic" (N=5745)		Assessment "not-purely somatic" (N= 1931)	
Therapeutic conversation				
No treatment recorded	32%		20%	
Reassuring	13%		24%	
Counselling (passive: therapeutic listening)	7%		18%	
Counselling (active: exploring)	9%		18%	
Information (on diagnosis)	27%		34%	
Information (on therapy)	31%		37%	
Health education	3%		5%	
Advice (stopping, restarting work)	1%		2%	
Medication				
No medication	56%		62%	
Psychotropic drugs				
- anxiolytics/hypnotics	.5%		1.8%	
- antidepressants	.0%	(2)	.2%	(3)
- other	2.6%		3.6%	
Mental health referral	-		.1%	(2)

Table 5.7 demonstrates again, something that has been mentioned earlier, the impact of an explicit psychological or social demand for help. In those cases where the general practitioner adds a "psychosocial footnote" to a physical diagnosis (which was almost by definition preceded by a physically based request for help), such an addendum has not much to say about the help offered.

Two further remarks need to be made with respect to treatment. In the first place, there is hardly any difference if we consider all physical complaints assessed as "not purely somatic" (points 2 - 5 on the 5-point scale on which the general practitioner assessed the psychosocial character of his diagnosis) or if we only consider the physical complaints assessed as "not purely psychological" and "purely psychological" (points 4 - 5 on the 5-point scale).

In the second place, there is no difference at all if we differentiate according to subjective and objective need, as we did before. It does not matter if a patient has experienced feelings of mental distress recently or if he scored above GHQ-threshold, the treatment of physical complaints with a psychosocial connotation for the general practitioner remains the same. The same is true for the physical diagnoses, considered as purely somatic by the general practitioner.

Conclusions

The repertoire of the general practitioner, as it is recorded on our registration forms, is rather a-specific and limited. We may summarize it briefly as follows;

In case of a psychological diagnosis, treatment consists of psychotropic drugs and counselling. In case of a social ICPC-diagnosis, counselling is the main kind of treatment. Somatic diagnoses with a psychosocial connotation receive some counselling, but significantly less than an explicit psychological or social diagnosis. In such cases hardly any psychotropic drugs are prescribed, neither are such patients referred to mental health specialists. To a lesser extent, the same can be said about psychological or social diagnoses resulting from a physical complaint. A great part of the psychosocial concerns of the general practitioner remains undiscussed when the patient's demands do not encourage such discussion or other kinds of psychosocial treatment. And, last but not least, the amount of treatment depends solely on the demand for psychosocial help and is independent from felt or normative need. The difference has already earlier been made, because patients with a "normative" need (high GHQ) have a much higher probability of consulting the general practitioner and expressing their psychosocial demands for help, thus receiving a psychological or social diagnosis, which in turn increases the probability of counselling, prescriptions and referral considerably.

The findings from earlier research (c.f. Goldberg and Huxley 1992, Giel, Koeter and Ormel 1990) that most patients with psychiatric diagnoses remain under the care of the general practitioner is confirmed. Only a small minority of patients with psychological and social problems (the latter being mostly relational problems) are referred. In case of physical diagnoses with a psychological assessment, a mental health referral is almost never observed (c.f. also Verhaak 1993).

The most important patient-characteristic influencing the kind of treatment is his or her age. Older patients receive less active counselling and more drug treatment. The probability of a referral is for them still less than it was already for younger patients.

Ormel et al. (1990) report comparable figures and a large difference between treatment of recognized patients (GHQ+/GP+) and unrecognized patients (GHQ+/GP-). A straight comparison is not possible, because our data concern episodes of illness instead of patients. However, a GHQ-positive patient with a physical diagnosis, assessed as purely somatic too, may be called an unrecognized patient. It seems only natural that these patients hardly receive any mental health treatment. The probability of receiving an anxiolytic or hypnotic for a physical diagnosis, assessed as purely somatic is more than three times lower than for a physical diagnosis, assessed as partly psychological, and tenfold less than for social or psychological diagnoses. The same is true for counselling and referral.

In Ormel's study mentioned above, recognized patients also appear to recover more than non-recognized patients. One difficulty in interpreting these results is the difference in initial scores between the recognized and non-recognized group, the former being more severely affected than the latter, according to their PSE-ID-score. The follow-up scores of both groups more or less equal result in further improvement for recognized patients. The finding that there was a rather weak or non-significant relationship between management by the general practitioner and outcome is important within the light of this chapter on management. The researchers suggest an important path between recognition and outcome, not mediated by management. In line with our results, we would draw attention for the fact that management is clearly related to the diagnostic label an episode is given. A psychological problem only comes on the agenda of doctor and patient when it has resulted in a psychosocial request for help, which in turn has been classified as a psychological or a social diagnosis in ICPC-terms. In such cases, doctor and patient seem to talk about the problem (given the high proportion counselling). These cases are the only ones in which the slight probability of more specialized help is at least considered. Non-Recognition as an assessment of a physical diagnosis excludes that consideration in advance, and diminishes the chances of counselling and drug prescribing too. Management of mental disorders presupposes psychological or social labelling of the problems presented.

Notes

1. **Table 5.8**

Treatment of patients with psychosocial diagnoses, with different preceding complaints (psychosocial vs not psychosocial)

	Psychosocial diagnosis preceded by psychosocial complaint	Psychosocial diagnosis not preceded by psychosocial complaint
Therapeutic conversation		
No treatment recorded	14%	17%
Reassuring	13%	29%
Counselling (passive: therapeutic listening)	46%	32%
Counselling (active: exploring)	52%	29%
Information (on diagnosis)	18%	34%
Information (on therapy)	18%	19%
Health education	3%	7%
Advice (stopping, restarting work)	10%	6%
Medication		
No medication	63%	75%
Psychotropic drugs	36%	16%
- anxiolytics/hypnotics	26%	10%
- antidepressants	9%	1%
- other	1%	5%
Referral/consultation		
Medical specialist	0.0%	4.5%
Mental Health	4.4%	1.6%
- psychiatrist	0.3%	0.4%
- mental health centre	1.8%	0.8%
- psychologist	0.5%	-
- social worker	1.8%	0.4%

6 Conclusion

Introduction

In the introductory chapter we asked ourselves if psychiatric epidemiological figures represented reality as people experience it. We have tried to demonstrate that such a normative need, at least as is expressed by epidemiological figures, provides only an incomplete picture. As was to be expected, we found a considerable gap between need according to psychiatric standards and felt need, expressed in a request for help. We proposed in our introduction three possible explanations for this divergence of needs and demands: either a lot of people suffer in terms of psychiatric standards, but do not share these standards, or a lot of people suffer and do not seek help, or a lot of people suffer but they are not recognized as suffering.

The following principal results of our study may contribute at the evaluation of these explanations:

- many people experience psychological distress and some of them are considered mentally disturbed by psychiatric standards. Only few people, considered mentally disturbed by psychiatric standards, do not experience feelings of distress. In general: normative need includes felt need but not vice versa
- although mentally distressed persons are more inclined to visit general practitioners (especially those who are indicated as distressed by psychiatric screening-instruments too), the majority do not see a general practitioner, at least not within a couple of months. A normative need leads in half of the cases to help seeking, a felt need to even fewer requests for help.
- although mentally distressed persons are more inclined to put forward demands for psychological help (especially those who arc indicated by psychiatric screening-instruments too), the great majority of them do not. Even if a professional carer is encountered, a normative need does not lead to a demand for help.

- psychosocial assessment by the general practitioner is not completely dependent on the nature of the demand for help: besides the demands for psychological and social help, demands formulated in general terms (pain, general unwell-being, fever, nausea) and neurological and digestive complaints are regularly assessed as being mainly psychosocial and even diagnosed within psychological categories
- psychosocial assessment by the general practitioner is dependent on patients' need on the one hand: patients, considered mentally disturbed by psychiatric standards have the highest probability of becoming assessed as "psychosocial", followed in this by patients who feel mentally distressed without reaching the psychiatric standard (although one third of the first group and half of the second group is still considered "purely somatic")
- on the other hand, patients who do not report feelings of mental distress are more easily assessed psychosocially when they are female, older or divorced. In other words: in case of "false positives" the general practitioner appears to be misguided by stereotypes.
- what is gained by general practitioner's recognition of physically presented signs of mental disorder is lost again by the fact that such symptoms are seldom treated with psychotherapy. Counseling, psychopharmacological treatment and mental health referral are mainly limited to psychological and social diagnoses, originating from a psychological or social demand for help.

Given our results we are inclined to make some amendments to the formulation of the explanation given above: A lot of people suffer according to psychiatric standards but their suffering is labelled differently, they seek different solutions and their doctors approve of it.

These amendments need a preamble before they can be put to the vote. This "preamble" can be centered around the following major themes:
- "they label it differently": mental disorder from different perspectives
- "they seek different solutions": the primacy of demand
- "doctors approve of it": the added value of general practitioner-judgement

In the next subchapters these subjects will be discussed respectively. When this has been done, it will be possible to come to conclusions about the presence of mental disorder and the contribution of medical care in general and especially what mental health care has to deliver in this respect. The last subchapter will be devoted to the consequences related to these conclusions.

Mental disorder from different perspectives

"People suffer according to a psychiatrist but people don't share these standards", we tried this as the first explanation for the discrepancy between normative need and the resulting demand for mental health treatment. To test this hypothesis normative needs and felt needs of patients were compared at population level.

Many people encounter problem situations and a lot of them experience feelings of emotional distress. A smaller number of them are also selected by objective screening-instruments because of the high probability of their having severe psychopathology. Subjective feelings of emotional distress exceed the objective indicators of it. Regarding the relationship between normative need and felt need we may conclude that psychiatrists do not assume disorder where the patient experiences no distress at all. The GHQ is not selecting people who report that they are in good health. Consequently, our first explanation is invalid. The great majority of people, indicated by the GHQ as potential cases of psychopathology are painfully aware of their distress and problematic situations. Nevertheless, some remarks need to be made.

Some categories of people are at a greater risk for all the kind of "needs" distinguished: women, the divorced, inhabitants of urbanized areas and the incapacitated or unemployed report more problem situations, feel worse and probably suffer more psychopathology than men, married people and the employed. The high risks of being "in need" in terms of professional standards is in line with the high risks in these categories of feeling disturbed in terms of their own experience.

Other categories experience more subjective feelings of distress without objectively running a greater risk than others: the elderly and the publicly-insured (lower socio-economic class) persons. Within these categories false positives might be expected. The opposite can also be found: widows/widowers have a higher risk of psychopathology but do not report more subjective feelings of distress than the married ones. They run a relatively high risk of not demanding help when they in fact are in need.

Education is a complicated characteristic: the least well-educated are most at risk of psychopathology and most frequently report feelings of emotional distress, but the most highly educated on the contrary report encountering more problem and stressful situations and record many more feelings of stress in their diary.

Furthermore, risk assessment becomes even more complicated because of different responding tendencies among different categories of respondents. We should ask ourselves to what extent the relations reported above represent "true relations". Mari and Williams (1986) conducted a validation study on the GHQ and compared scores on the GHQ-12 with the outcome of the Clinical Interview Schedule. There were more false negatives among males than among females and more false positives among the less well-educated than among the more highly educated. This means that a relatively large number of men scored below threshold on the GHQ-12 but appeared mentally disturbed during the psychiatric interview. The opposite was true for the less well-educated: a relatively large number of them score above GHQ-threshold but did not appear to be a case of mental illness during the clinical interview. Misclassification, according to Mari and Williams, should not necessarily imply error in the questionnaire.

> Thus, the source of misclassification may be located within the respondent as well as within the questionnaire. According to this interpretation, the false negative respondents can be regarded as underestimating their psycho-emotional symptoms .... and false positive respondents as maximizing them .... They therefore represent two different aspects of illness behaviour and sociodemographic factors may play an important role in influencing it (Mari and Williams 1986, p.376).

In this view, it remains debatable whether women, the divorced, the unemployed, and the incapacitated are more "in need" or only expressing their "need" better in terms of the GHQ, while men, married people and the employed are underestimating their psycho-emotional symptoms. Although the higher case-load among the former groups is corroborated by their higher probability of reporting problem situations and feelings of mental distress, this may be a result of the same mechanism of maximizing psycho-emotional symptoms. In the following we shall observe that for most of these groups this may indeed be considered an aspect of illness behaviour.

Apart from differences between respondents in their tendency to complain, general health feeling of the respondents may influence GHQ-scores also. In an earlier paper (Bensing and Verhaak 1994) it was concluded that patients with a high GHQ-score reported more somatic complaints, more chronic somatic conditions and a feeling of inferior general health than patients with a low GHQ-score. Moreover, they consulted far more medical specialists, physiotherapists and alternative healers, they consumed more medication and had more days sick-leave. This kind of result leads to renewed attention to Dohrenwendt's criticism of the GHQ and similar instruments, which may indicate not psychopathology but general feelings of helplessness, for instance caused by ill-health feelings. At least we may conclude from our study that these feelings of helplessness exceed the ordinary feelings of emotional distress, as the latter seem a necessary but not sufficient condition for the former.

Moreover, in this respect, the role of health status in the help seeking process is an interesting one. In the absence of feelings of distress or an objective need (high GHQ) help seeking is determined by the subjective health perception of the patient, his acute somatic complaints and the number of chronic conditions he is suffering from. Putting it in a simplistic way: patients without a felt or normative need for psychological help visit their general practitioner because they are ill. (see also: van der Zee, 1982).

People who seem disturbed according to objective psychiatric standards, the GHQ+ patients (who also experience subjective feelings of distress), do not consult their general practitioner because of their acute symptoms or chronic conditions. At least, these aspects of health status do not differentiate between those who consult the general practitioner and those who do not. The only health status variable of any importance in this respect is the subjective health perception. Their background characteristics which determine help seeking - female, no paid employment, publicly-insured - are not affected by controlling for health status. Simplifying again, people with an normative need consult their general practitioner irrespective of their health status, but more easily when they are in the possession of the characteristics mentioned (Verhaak, in press).

Thus, we may conclude that patients, indicated by the GHQ as being in need in terms of psychiatric standards, feel helpless. Some of them will be psychiatric cases, some of them will be characterized by a tendency to complain without being real psychiatric cases. The subjective feeling of helplessness may be the direct result of psychiatric illness, but may also result from physical conditions and bad health.

Given this "mer à boire" of possible interpretations, we assume that most people who are indicated as "cases", recognize their subjective feeling of being unwell and tend to seek medical help, but do not view themselves as potential psychiatric clients. Evidence for this assumption stems from our analysis of help seeking behaviour and the complaints and symptoms brought forward during those consultations. With only half of all "cases" visiting their general practitioner in a three month period, and one sixth of them expressing complaints of a psychosocial nature, we arrive at the conclusion: a lot of people suffer in terms of psychiatric standards -and a lot more suffer as well without reaching the psychiatric level - but they give a different meaning to their feelings.

Our analysis of general practitioner's psychological and social diagnoses presents the next field of tension between two perspectives: normative need according to the general practitioner and normative need according to psychiatry.

The incidences and prevalences, reported in chapter 4, (table 4.9) indeed show that the psychiatric taxonomy in general is not very suitable for general practice. Conspicuous features of diagnoses made by general practitioners are the predominance of symptom diagnoses and the high prevalence/incidence ratio of the most frequently made diagnoses, anxiety, sleeping disorder and depression. The prevalence rate of these diagnoses is twenty-six (sleeping disorder) to four times as high as the incidence rate, to a considerable extent due to repeat prescriptions. This suggests a kind of hard core of patients, regularly visiting their general practitioner with well-known psychological or social symptoms. The diagnostic picture does not correspond very well with the results from the American Epidemiological Catchment Area study, discussed in chapter 3, providing a picture of the population in DSM-III terminology.

From the ECA-study we know the one year prevalence of specific DSM-III diagnoses in the American population. We have noticed already in the discussion of chapter 4 that it is not simply possible to extrapolate our three-month prevalences to year prevalences. We may however assume that our year prevalence is somewhere between one and four times our three-month prevalence. Table 6.1 presents some prevalences next to one another.

Table 6.1
Prevalences from ECA (population) and current study (GP-diagnosis) (percentages)

Diagnosis	ECA	Current study
Phobia	8.8	.2 - .8
Alcohol abuse/dependence	6.3	.1 - .5
Generalized anxiety	3.8	.1 - .3
Major depression	3.7	-
Neurotic depression	-	1.1 - 4.4
Drug abuse/dependence	2.5	.1 - .3
Cognitive impairment	5.0	.02 - .06
Antisocial personality	1.2	-
Obsessive compulsive	1.7	-
Schizophrenia	1.0	.1 - .2
Anxious, nervous	-	2.6 - 10.4
Sleeping disorder	-	2.7 - 10.7
Overwork	-	.8 - 3.6
Stress	-	.6 - 2.3
Tension headache	-	.4 - 1.5
Hyperventilation syndrome	-	.4 - 1.4

Comparing the ECA prevalences with our prevalences we can conclude in the first place that most of the ECA-disorders with a prevalence of 1% or more are hardly diagnosed by primary care physicians. The most striking example is phobia, with a prevalence of 8.8% in the ECA study and a three month prevalence of .2% in our study. Cognitive impairments, antisocial personality, and obsessive/compulsive behaviour, all more than 1% prevalent in the ECA study are scarcely diagnosed. Addiction problems and schizophrenia are about five times more prevalent in the ECA study than in our highest estimate.

That leaves us with depression and anxiety. Major depressive episodes have in the ECA study a one-year prevalence of 3.7%. Neurotic depression in our study, which has much less severe criteria, is estimated at between 1.1% and 4.4%. It seems probable that depression in general is underestimated too, compared with American data. Anxiety leaves us with an interesting case. The ECA study reports a prevalence rate of generalized anxiety of 3.8%. If we confine ourselves in our study to anxiety disorder we can report a range between .1% and .3%. If we are allowed, however, to include feelings of anxiousness and nervousness, we arrive at the much higher range of 2.7% to 10.8%.

Furthermore, there are a number of typical primary care diagnoses, not known in the DSM-III, to be added. Sleeping disorder (2.7% - 10.7%), overwork (.8% - 3.6%), stress (.6% - 2.3%), tension headache (.4% - 1.5%) and the hyperventilation syndrome (.4% - 1.4%) are prevalent diagnoses in general practice. Incidentally, keeping the foregoing discussion in mind, there might be a lot of misclassified depression among the latter symptom-diagnoses.

Another category of psychosocial distress, not classifiable in the DSM-III, but frequently encountered by family physicians, are the relational and working problems, and the emotional problems associated with illness and death of family members. Taken together they have a prevalence of .7% - 2.8% of the practice population on a yearly basis.

In short, a psychiatrical category system does not seem the most appropriate way of classifying mental problems encountered in primary care. The picture which emerges from general practice looks more like a rather disorganized collection of symptoms, pointing mainly to anxiety and depression, with some stress and addiction among it. Many of these symptoms are found within the two dimensions of neuroses, proposed by Goldberg et al. (1987) and later elaborated by Goldberg and Huxley (1992). Except that a great number of the recorded symptom diagnoses refer to only two dimensions, anxiety and depression, both dimensions proved to be highly interrelated too. Goldberg et al. conclude from these results that

> the poor agreement between general practitioners and psychiatrists for these common disorders .... reflects the fact that the patients do not form themselves into natural groupings (Goldberg et al. 1987, p.468).

This interpretation is in keeping with the model proposed by Foulds, discussed in chapter 1: On the lowest level of his hierarchical system a common core of affective symptoms occurs in a number of mood disturbances. It is also comparable with Terluin's (1994) results for primary care (cf chapter 4): all patients with psychosocial problems report a-specific distress symptoms but only a (small) part of them add "real" neurotic symptoms to it. In other words: many people suffer from a-specific symptoms to which no further diagnosis can be attached. Such mood disturbances are the far most prevalent psychological disorders and women, elderly and the less well-educated are mostly affected by them.

From such a comparison between need as DSM-III defines it and need as general practitioners diagnose it, we conclude that patients in general practice are suffering from a number of symptoms from which psychiatric diagnoses **can** be distilled. However, such diagnoses suggest a surplus value a general practitioner is unwilling to attach to it. It may be incompetence, for a general practitioner is not a qualified psychiatric diagnostician. It may, however also be connected with the importance attached by general practitioners to the demand for help. For instance, many patients ask for a prescription, resulting in the diagnosis "sleeping disturbance"; a general practitioner may react: "if that women ..." -mostly they are elderly women- " wants a sleeping pill, why not give it to her?". It may also be connected with the poor therapeutic prospects of a full-blown psychiatric diagnosis.

A last comment on the relationship between different perspectives may be made on the fact that important patient categories for the most frequently made diagnoses anxious / depressive / sleeping disorder are older publicly insured women, categories who were on the population level more at risk as regards feelings of mental distress than for psychopathology, as indicated by the GHQ. For such groups, a picture emerges of a group, well known to the general practitioner, with worries and concerns that come with age, who can manage on that level without a need for psychiatric intervention.

The primacy of demand

"People do suffer indeed, but they seek other than psychiatric solutions", was our second amendment.

Whether they have feelings of helplessness or probable psychopathology, people with an elevated GHQ-score at least appear to be the most severe cases. These persons enter the official medical circuit more frequently and with a clearer demand for psychological help than those who just express feelings of emotional distress without a high GHQ-score. It has been illustrated in a lot of ways: The odds on consulting a general practitioner are higher, in case of such a consultation the GHQ+ patient has more than double the likelihood of presenting a psychosocial demand for help than a patient who just "feels" distressed, and later they have a much better chance of getting their somatic demands translated into a psychosocial assessment by the general practitioner.

This should however, not divert our attention from the fact that half of these patients, who are "objectively" in need of help choose not to seek help at all within the medical sector, at least not within the limited period of three months. In general, the majority of people reporting feelings of distress do not consult a medical doctor within three months, probably because they have better solutions for their problems. And again, patient characteristics play a role.

Some people have a higher probability of contacting a general practitioner than others. Irrespective of their psychological condition men and those in employment have a lower probability than women and people without paid employment (incapacitated, unemployed, housewives/-men, retired); in case of probable psychopathology the publicly-insured also have better chances than privately-insured of meeting a general practitioner. In case of feelings of distress without psychopathology the less well-educated have better chances than the more highly educated.

Most of the characteristics enabling help-seeking behaviour are also determinants for the subjective or objective need, as established at population level. Thus, women have a greater probability of mental disorder, but in case they are in distress, there is also a greater probability that they will seek help than men. The same goes for the unemployed or incapacitated. This may improve the probability of detection for women, unemployed or incapacitated. If detection of mental distress might be called an advantage, these people are doubly blessed. On the other hand, men, people in paid employment and the privately-insured are less prone to be mentally disturbed, but where they are, they are behind women, those not employed or publicly-insured in their chances of being detected by a general practitioner: they have a double disadvantage.

This mechanism does not work, however, for the divorced or widows/widowers. Although they experience relatively frequent feelings of distress, and are more often indicated by the GHQ as probable cases of mental illness, their chance of a doctor's consultation, when in distress, are equal to those of married or unmarried people.

Need is rarely translated in a direct demand for help. Only seven per cent of all reasons for consultation can be considered psychological or social, most of the reasons are feelings of anxiety and depression, sleep disturbances, stress reactions and problems in the working or relational situation. Of course, the majority of patients did not indicate a sense of need, either subjective or objective. But of those who did, only fifteen to thirty per cent put forward psychosocial complaints or other reasons for encounter directly.

The expectation that most demands for psychosocial help would be put forward by women, the unemployed and incapacitated and the fewest by men and people in paid employment proved not to be the case. In fact, neither with respect to sex, nor to employment status could significant differences in presentation of psychosocial complaints be found. They were to be found, however, with respect of age and marital status. Divorced people in particular and the oldest age-group presented a relatively large number of psychosocial complaints. In these cases the distribution of psychosocial demands more or less represents the distribution of subjective and objective needs. Another explanation needs to be sought for the lack of the relationships mentioned earlier.

Maybe this explanation can be found in the presentation of physical complaints, reformulated by the general practitioner in his diagnostic process into a psychological or social diagnosis. Psychological diagnoses not only result from psychological complaints but relatively often from general complaints like fatigue, pain or general feeling of being unwell, digestive and neurological complaints. In this context we see a majority of women. Their expected predominance in psychosocial demands is translated in physical rather than in psychological terms. It can thus only been made visible after detection and "translation" by the general practitioner, the subject of our next section. On the other hand, the physical complaints of patients without paid employment are not disproportionally translated by the general practitioner into psychosocial diagnoses.

Anticipating the following subsections, it should already be remarked here that, although the general practitioners adds a substantial number of psychosocial assessments to those cases which were already psychosocial in terms of the demand for help, they lose this gain again by not attaching any psychotherapeutic consequences to it. Hence, the primacy of demand.

How should we evaluate a situation in which only a minority of the felt and normative need is translated into a demand for psychological help, such a demand being almost a necessary condition for psychotherapeutic treatment?

We could take the stand that the patient is a competent medical consumer. The patient is the expert on his own experience and qualified to demand what he needs.

Emotional distress is a rather common experience for a patient, and in most cases they seem perfectly able to deal with it themselves. Three eighths of the population experience feelings of psychological distress and only 40% of them consult a general practitioner. The great majority of these visitors (85%) did not express any psychosocial demand for help.

It has been argued (Lamberts 1991) that general practitioners should not assume that the problems, brought forward by the patient are essentially different from what they "really want". Doctors should not consider the patient's reason for visit as a metaphor for "the real reason". This point stresses the above interpretation of the patient as a competent medical consumer.

Taking the patient's demand as sort of a gold standard, psychosocial problems in primary care constitute a minor part of the total amount of problems presented in general practice. From this point of view, general practitioners magnify the size of the problem unnecessarily by assessing one third of the patients consulting them during a three month period as having non-somatic problems, whereas only fifteen per cent have expressed a psychosocial demand for help. Serious debates have been held in the Netherlands regarding this stance. (Lamberts and Hofmans-Okkes versus Tielens 1993).

Contrary to this argumentation are the contact frequencies of patients who report feelings of distress, their requests for repeat prescriptions, and the psychotropic medication given to them. In all cases this is ten to fifty per cent more than for patients without feelings of distress. This indicates that these patients in fact express more psychosocial problems by their behaviour than in their direct demands for help. In other words: taking the patient as a yardstick leads to an underestimation of mental illness in general practice. The general practitioner should detect these hidden psychological disorders and treat the real causes of unexplained somatic complaints. This recommendation, however, though simply stated in seventeen words, might prove to be the quintessence of general practitioners' problems with primary mental health care. Because, treatment of such disorder requires exactly that understanding in the character of the disorder that is lacking in most patients, as we have argued before. It remains debatable if such an understanding, and in consequence a shift in interpretation of complaints with a resulting motivation for treatment can be achieved.

In this respect a number of experiments can be reported in which psychiatrists offered consultation services to general practitioners and patients with physical complaints without a somatic explanation for it. Katon et al. (1990) reported such an intervention to increase the prescription of antidepressants, without however having any effect on the psychiatric status of the patient. Smith, Monson and Ray (1986) reported a successful intervention in patients with somatizing disorder. Patients with somatization disorder in terms of the DSM-III constitute a highly selected sample from the much larger group of patients, seen by the general practitioner each day, with unexplained somatic complaints.

In a pilot study, examining the feasibility of psychiatric consultation, we concluded that general practitioners were willing to ask for a consultation for about twenty per cent of patients with complaints without a possible somatic explanation. Those patients who were selected for such a consultation appeared to be more convinced about the role psychological factors were playing than the eighty per cent with unexplained somatic complaints who were not selected. (Collijn et al. 1994). Such evidence suggests that in some cases it is possible to offer treatment to patients who do not demand psychosocial help while they need it. However only those patients could be selected who had a favourable attitude towards a psychological explanation of their complaints. Not much evidence has been found about its reach or its efficacy.

Hence, most people who suffer in terms of psychiatric standards seek solutions other than psychiatric ones: they rarely put forward requests for psychological help, and yet such a request is considered a necessary condition for a successful psychotherapeutic intervention. This situation also explains the somehow paradoxical results around recognition and treatment of psychological distress by general practitioners, which we will pay attention to in the following section.

The added value of general practitioner-judgments?

Patients in general recognize their problems but do not consider themselves in need of psychiatric treatment and hence seek non-psychiatric solutions for their problems. "And doctors approve of it, we added as third amendment. The general practitioner plays an intermediary role in this process. On the one hand, the general practitioner has to take psychological factors into account when making a diagnosis. On the other hand, he should take into account the possibilities for treatment at his disposal. Possibilities that are in turn heavily dependent on the demand of the patient.

Recognition is not such a problem in case of a psychological or social demand. The problem is clear in that case and that situation provides opportunities for treatment. Unfortunately, psychosocial problems are not always expressed in such a straightforward manner. More than 90% of all requests are put in physical terms, but less than 70% are assessed by the general practitioner as being purely somatic. Recognition by the general practitioner of the psychological aspects behind physically presented complaints is critical in many cases.

Some interesting results about recognition are reported. In the first place, the recognition rate increases with the subjective (felt) and objective (normative) need of the patient. When need according to the objective standard has been assessed, the odds on psychosocial assessment are twice as high as in the case of absence of objective or subjective need. On the other hand, taking absolute numbers into account, half of all people with a psychosocial assessment by the general practitioner have no need at all and one third of the people with both objective and subjective needs did not have any psychosocial assessment during their contacts. But to a certain extent, general practitioners appear sensitive to the GHQ-status of patients and to their subjective feelings as well.

A second area of interest to be mentioned here, are the patient characteristics influencing psychosocial assessments by the general practitioner. This influence seems mediated by the objective or subjective need of the patient. In absence of GHQ-caseness most of the patient characteristics are related to the general practitioner-assessment as "non-somatic". These patients, from a psychiatrist's view false positives, are more easily assessed as "not somatic" if they are female, middle-aged, divorced or without paid employment. On the other hand, from those scoring high on the GHQ, only the less well-educated are easily picked out by the general practitioner as having non-somatic diagnoses. In the former case, stereotyping plays a certain role.

Here we are in the middle of the discussion about the ability of the general practitioner to recognize psychological disorders. Following the line of reasoning we have maintained throughout this book, we should first ask, recognition of which psychological disorders: the patients' manifest feelings of distress, disorders as defined by the professional standard or the explicit demands put forward by the patient.

As has been remarked already, the latter is not the problem we are dealing with. The only difficulty related to the demand is our impression that demand is really an underestimation of the real psychological (normative) need.

The group of patients with feelings of distress without an normative need for which no explicit demand for help has been formulated do not seem to be the problem either. The fact that a patient recognizes these feelings without attaching a request for help to them seems to indicate that they are transient feelings for which other solutions have already been found by the patient. The moderate impact of these feelings on help-seeking behaviour strengthens us in this view. In these cases we might really speak of the patient as a competent medical consumer. Thus, it seems reasonable to limit ourselves in this discussion to the non-recognized GHQ-cases who pair this objective need with feelings of distress.

It has been remarked that a distressed patient, consulting his general practitioner, may also consult him for a purely physical reason, not related at all to his mental condition (Bensing and Beerendonk 1990), or that non-detected patient at the moment of screening might be detected in follow-up contacts (Giel, Koeter and Ormel 1990). However, our results in this respect have been found on an aggregated level. We are not talking about non-recognition during one particular consultation. On the contrary: our non-recognized GHQ-cases did not have any psychological assessment during several months.

These false negatives, people scoring positively on the GHQ without being assessed as psychological by the general practitioner are the problem, many have been troubled with. As we have seen, this non-recognition is mainly due to a physical presentation of complaints. Katon et al. (1986) suggest that somatization and co-morbidity result in an underestimate of psychiatric illness by screening questionnaires which are primarily psychological in focus. Our findings, however, that the majority of persons, detected by such a screening questionnaire (GHQ), still stuck to physical complaints when seeing their general practitioner, contradicts this result. Somatization and co-morbidity may however be important causes for non-recognition.

As was mentioned earlier, people scoring high on the GHQ report more chronic conditions and acute symptoms than people below threshold (Bensing and Verhaak 1994). Schulberg, McClelland and Burns (1987) distinguish among the several ways in which co-morbidity of depressive and medical disorders can manifest itself. Depression is, in addition to anxiety, the major psychological disorder within primary care. Both depression and anxiety combine mood and neurovegetative symptoms and lend themselves therefore to confusion of physical and mental illness. For these reasons, depression might serve as pars pro toto. The manifestations of co-morbidity in this case are the following:

Physical symptoms of depression Highly prevalent complaints in masked depression are pain, musculoskeletal, neurological, gastro-intestinal and cardio-pulmonary complaints. In Schulberg's words: "depression mimics medical disorder". These physical manifestations of depression, a typical psychobiological syndrome, might mislead the general practitioner by their physical appearance.

Depressive symptoms of medical illness Symptomatology of organic conditions may mimic depression as well. Schulberg et al. enumerate an extensive number of diseases, pertaining to most bodily systems, which might generate depressive symptoms. As a result, a physician will have to be vigilant in accepting depressive symptoms at their face value, possibly resulting in non-recognition.

Depressive reactions to medical illness Impairment induced by a medical disorder might cause a depressive reaction. Furthermore, depression might occur simultaneously with an unrelated medical disorder. The mechanisms of the latter sort have been sought in psychodynamic and psychophysiological explanations, but they are not clear yet. Nevertheless, the physical symptoms may obscure the presence of depression and cause trouble for the diagnosing physician.

Regarding the assessment of whether physical symptoms constitute a mood disorder and whether mood symptoms possibly belie organic pathology, the review of Schulberg et al. is rather pessimistic. Findings concerning biomedical tests are called ambiguous, while psychological tests suffer from the confounding meaning of items assessing physical symptoms. The latter especially yields different results, depending on the population to which they are applied, somatic items appear insensitive in chronically ill populations. In fact the psychological tests reviewed have only limited value in distinguishing functional disorders and medical illness.

Still another explanation of massive non-recognition when patients limit themselves to somatic complaints and symptoms might be the severity of these patients' mental disorder. "Somatizers" and "psychologizers" have been compared in a number of studies.

Bridges et al. (1991) defined somatization using the following criteria:

- the patient seeks help for somatic manifestations of psychiatric illness without presenting psychological symptoms;
- the patient attributes these somatic manifestations to physical illness;
- symptoms must justify a psychiatric diagnosis according to the standard research criteria;
- research psychiatrist must be convinced that treatment of the psychiatric disorder would cause the somatic symptoms to disappear.

Psychologizers were patients who presented psychological symptoms to the doctor. Somatizers were found to be similar to psychologizers in many respects (sociodemographic, personality) but they were less depressed, reported lower levels of social dissatisfaction, social stress and less dependence on their relatives, had a more unsympathetic attitude towards mental illness and had been more treated as medical in-patients in the past. In other words, they were less severely ill and had a negative attitude towards a psychological demands for help.

Wright (1990) compared patients presenting with psychological symptoms in general practice with patients presenting with somatic symptoms for which no physical explanation was evident at the time of consultation. The latter had lower scores on severity of psychiatric distress, fewer individual symptoms and fewer severe symptoms than the former.

In our own research (Verhaak and Tijhuis 1994) a similar comparison was made with the same results. Moreover, during a one year follow-up of the two groups of patients, three quarter of the somatizing patients did not present somatic symptoms again without a physical explanation nor with psychological symptoms. They remained, however, frequent attenders, but mostly with symptoms assessed by the general practitioner as purely somatic.

These three studies provide evidence that (the frequently unrecognized) disturbed patients with physical symptomatology are in many cases in a less severe condition than patients with a psychological demand.

To conclude our discussion of non-recognition: people who mask their psychological distress by somatic requests for help may be the less severe sufferers who are considered mentally disturbed in psychiatric terms. General practitioners tend to follow the somatic interpretation of the patient in their management of the disorder, even when they recognize the psychological background of the complaints. This primacy of the patient's demand for help is also illustrated by the diagnoses, made by the general practitioner.

For several reasons therefore physical symptoms of disturbed patients in our research might have been assessed as purely somatic. However, exactly those physical symptoms, mentioned by Schulberg et al., that are associated with depression have been observed by us as leading frequently to a psychological diagnosis. Maybe the general practitioners have missed a lot too, but in each case they seem to be aware of the significance of symptoms like pain, headache, and abdominal complaints.

Moreover, this awareness has lead to a considerable higher identification rate of psychosocial problems than could be expected on the basis of patient's demand. While 7% of the patients put forward psychosocial complaints, 18% have been diagnosed at least once within the ICPC-categories Psyche or Social and 32% of the complaints have been assessed as being not purely somatic.

The interesting point, possibly a point for action, is what we called the lost gain of the general practitioner. A number of patients, presenting with the symptoms of depression like abdominal pain, neurological complaints and musculoskeletal symptoms are recognized as "possibly psychosocial", but this assessment has no implications for treatment. In other words: general practitioners seem to approve to the decision of the patient to avoid a psychological interpretation of their complaints. Only psychosocial diagnoses resulting from psychosocial complaints lead to psychosocial treatment. This is, where the question mark in the title "the added value of recognition by the general practitioner?" comes from. Even if the recognition problem is solved, the ensuing behaviour remains problematic, given the nature of primary health care, expectations of patients and limitations of the ten minute consultation.

Conclusions

"A lot of people are suffering in terms of psychiatric standards but not all of them share these standards, many of them seek different solutions and general practitioners often seem to approve of such decisions". This is the statement we have defended over the last few pages. What consequences may this new outlook have?

All parties involved, patients, general practitioners and psychiatrists should draw conclusions. They can be drawn at the level of psychiatric epidemiology, at the level of the process of primary health care and at the level of population-oriented mental health education.

At the epidemiological level attention should be given to the large number of patients presumably in need but not demanding any help. Partly because they can cope with their problems, partly because they do not consider themselves as having a psychological problem and, most important, partly because they do not see a reasonable chance of solving their problems.

At the level of the doctor-patient interaction in primary care research efforts and new developments are needed to provide primary care doctors with suitable interventions. This being fulfilled, attention is needed for better communication techniques in order to recognize those patients who could benefit from interventions. And last but not least, general practitioners should be taught to express their suspicions of psychological origins for the complaints.

This fits in with the last level at which action might be needed. The general public should be informed better about the possibilities general practitioners have, to help them cope with problematic situations, or perhaps even about options for successful intervention.

We shall dwell on these three topics more comprehensively in the last three sections.

Epidemiological consequences: Mental disorder from a mental health services perspective

Our concern with the weight attached to psychiatric epidemiological figures stems from the linkage which has been laid between such a normative need, as we have called it throughout this book and the use which should been made of mental health services by these patients.

Were the assessment of psychiatric need in the population only meant to describe the population, just as a population can be described in terms of the presence of certain religions, cultural views or political votes, it would offer another piece of information, mainly of academic interest. But of course it is not. Assessment of psychiatric need in the population serves the honourable goal of detecting shortcomings in the current system of care delivery, enabling the planning of services and possibly developing prevention programs. This is the way community surveys, following the Goldberg and Huxley model, are meant and interpreted. To paraphrase our citation of Leighton in the beginning: community surveyors expect agreement among psychiatrists that the individuals detected in their studies are psychiatric cases who need treatment.

This is the right point to recall the discussion in chapter 1 about psychiatric classification. Based on characteristics of clinical populations symptoms have been selected by which categories of psychiatric disorder are defined. One important characteristic of those patients from whom these definitions are borrowed is by definition lacking in the population at large, i.e.: the fact that clinical help has been sought and provided. Checking symptoms in a population where no actual demand for help exists leads to a number of symptoms being put together to constitute a totally different "Sum of Parts" or "Gestalt" than the same symptoms presented in a clinical population where a demand for help has been put forward. Because, related to the actual demand for help there are other features, like lack of support and feelings that things are unbearable.

In our opinion a more integrated picture is needed to determine the amount of treatment needed. As we said in the introduction: knowledge about diseases (which equals "normative need") is necessary but not sufficient to understand the epidemiology of human suffering and problem solving. In this picture the normative need, as a psychiatrist would record it is indispensable, a fact which has also become clear in our study. In addition, however, more attention should be paid to the actual urgency for treatment, given the circumstances of the patient and the treatment options. It is recommended to distinguish in population surveys between normative needs in an academic sense and normative needs which constitute "suitable cases for treatment".

Almost all patients who were in need according to psychiatric standards also felt mentally distressed themselves. The tendency to seek help among these persons was considerably greater than it was among those who felt distressed without fulfilling the professional criteria.

The other side of the coin is the help-seeking behaviour of those patients in absolute figures. Half of those who should consult a psychiatrist did not even feel the urge to consult a general practitioner. As there are hardly any barriers, financial or geographical, to so doing, we are inclined to conclude that not everybody who is in need in the eyes of a psychiatrist is convinced of the use of seeking medical help. From a point of view in which need and health services use are linked, it is useful to distinguish those needs for which a treatment is available. If the patient does not consider it worthwhile seeking medical treatment himself, there is a problem in this respect. A minority of needs, such as psychotic disorders, but also anti-social behaviour, can be assessed by an outsider, and the request for treatment in such cases will usually come from outsiders too. However, most patients who are in need according to professionals, are considered as such because of their own reports and if they do not conclude from their experience that they need professional help, treatment is very difficult to offer.

If we continue along this path, we must conclude that if medical help is sought, the demand for help rarely explicitly concerns psychological problems. Here, we are confronted with at least two problems. Failure of the general practitioner to recognize some of the patients who appear in need in terms of psychiatric standards is such a problem. We come back at this problem in the next section. A lack of treatment possibilities is the second problem, probably as large as the first one. As far as the mental health services approach is concerned, it should be noticed that normative needs, not combined with a demand for psychosocial help, should only been taken into consideration if an effective treatment can be offered. As far as epidemiology is concerned, this is the major point to be stressed: epidemiological figures sec (i.e. the normative needs) are of only academic interest. To be useful for mental health care developments (like planning of services, training capacity), inclusion of treatment possibilities, linked with demand for treatment is essential.

In the following section we shall discuss developments and possible new ways for primary care to cope with these problems.

Possible consequences for primary mental health care

Recognition problem

The problem of non-recognition is closely related to the tendency of those in need to present with only physical complaints and symptoms. As a consequence, they receive somatic treatment for problems which are essentially psychosocial, even when they are recognized by the general practitioner as patients with psychosocial problems. Psychotherapeutic approaches are not possible, unless the patient accepts a different interpretation, something most doctors do not even attempt.

Although many of the somatizers may not be in the most severe state of mental illness, they generate high costs in health care, they are time consuming and frustrating patients to the general practitioner, and recognition appears to be a means of breaking through the vicious circle. A number of suggestions has been made to improve recognition by the general practitioner.

Schulberg and Burns (1988) recommend "research on why rather than whether hidden psychiatric morbidity occurs". It has been sufficiently established that a lot of psychiatric morbidity remains unrecognized. Clinical decision making in primary care practice and patient physician interaction that facilitate or hinder diagnostic accuracy should be the focus of investigation. In their earlier paper on co-morbidity (Schulberg, McClelland and Burns 1987), the biopsychosocial model, developed by Engel is advocated. This model is considered particularly relevant to the diagnosis of somatization which requires consideration of biomedical data as well as psychiatric and sociocultural information. In fact such a research line has been developed within the Netherlands institute of primary care, where videotaped doctor-patient interactions have been studied in order to determine conversation styles which facilitate detection of psychological disorders (Bensing 1991a, 1991b, 1992, 1994, Verhaak 1986, 1988; cf. also Marks, Golberg and Hillier 1979). Important qualities of a conversation style adapted to the detection and treatment of psychological complaints appear to be the affective behaviour of the general practitioner (showing empathy and attention) and patient-centered behaviour. Affective behaviour not only contributed to the psychosocial quality of the consultation as assessed by a panel of experienced general practitioners but it was also the principal determinant of the biomedical quality.

Another possibility might be the provision of feedback by screening lists to the general practitioner. Giel, Koeter and Ormel (1990) conclude that the literature is ambivalent about the effects of such an intervention. They propose that the general practitioner's awareness of the nature and prevalence of mental health problems, as well as the existence of high risk groups should be increased. In this respect we should point to the results mentioned above, which showed that general practitioners are in fact informed about the existence of high risk groups, to such an extent that in the absence of objective disorder they tend to wrongly attribute mental disorder to these groups.

Goldberg and Bridges (1987) at last argue in favour of a taxonomy of neurosis which better fits the situation in general practice, where an unbroken continuum between states of normality and mood disorder is encountered. But this brings us to the following section.

Treatment problem

An onset to the linkage between need and treatment has been given by Goldberg. In a number of papers, Goldberg (1992) has argued that a general practitioner does not benefit at all from a mere classification, be it in dimensions or categories. He is much better served with a classification according to the required interventions. In this respect, four groups of patients are distinguished.

Disorders requiring recognition and discussion Included in this group are transient disorders and those at the threshold of "caseness". Goldberg considers mild anxiety/depressive disorders and somatization (cf. Bridges et al.1991) to this category. These patients need recognition and restoration of hope. Important skills for the general practitioner are the ability to recognize disorder and to discuss the social and interpersonal setting. In case of somatization a general practitioner needs to be able to re-attribute the patient's somatic symptoms.

Patients requiring support and social intervention "Chronic neuroses", patients with long standing disorders, which may well include chronic physical illness as well as non-psychotic psychological symptoms. Frequent attenders with frequent psychotropic drug use, often known as problem patients, causing sinking feelings. These patients should not be labelled as mentally ill; instead they should learn other coping behaviours. Important skills for the general practitioner are an ability to tolerate the patient not getting better, a continued monitoring of the patient's social adjustment and physical health and a timely for social help. Manifold prescription of different drugs which keep patients dependent and wrongly convinced that their problems can be resolved by psychotropics is contra-indicated.

Disorders which require specific interventions Disorders which fulfil research characteristics and for which a medical or behavioural treatment of proven value exists, such as schizophrenia, mania, severe depressive illness (including depressed somatizers), phobic illnesses, obsessive-compulsive disorders, anxiety states and sexual disorders. General practitioners should be able to assess the severity of these illnesses and, in case of depression, make rational decisions about the prescription of anti-depressants. The most important skill in all groups, however is a good counselling technique.

Distress not helped by detection In Goldberg's view, this is a small group of patients who are defensive and in fact have visited the doctor for something else. They will not benefit by intruding in their privacy.

Goldberg's classification is recognition of the fact that a lot of mentally distressed primary care attenders are not to be diagnosed within DSM-III categories of psychiatric illness. Patients with a "classic" psychiatric diagnosis belong to Goldberg's third group. It remains hard to decide, however, to what extent the symptoms of mood disorders, so frequently encountered, belong to the group of borderlines, requiring attention and discussion, or to the group of problem patients. Secondly, it depends more or less on the faith one has in general medicine, if one classifies the majority of the diagnoses made by the general practitioners in our study in the first category, or if one considers them as unrecognized disorders requiring specific interventions.

As a classification of our data in Goldberg's system is not possible a posteriori, a direct evaluation of the treatment given cannot be based on his criteria. Nevertheless, we shall consider our results about management in the light of these comments.

What treatment should be offered according to Goldberg? To patients requiring recognition and discussion, active counselling, eventually paired with listening and reassuring forms of therapeutic conversation are of importance. In cases of somatizing patients who are sufficiently depressed, antidepressants may be considered, otherwise drug prescription is not considered necessary.

In case of patients requiring social support and social interventions, passive forms of counselling and medical monitoring might be expected, eventually with a referral to social work. Drugs should be avoided.

Disorders which require specific interventions are to be referred to psychiatry or psychology departments; anti-depressant therapy and specialized counselling techniques, directed at behavioural change might be expected.

What did we find actually? Too much prescription of anxiolytics and hypnotics presumably. From the great number of repeat prescriptions within this category we may conclude that probably a significant part of them served as a mere palliative for patients who would have been better off with a minimum of drugs. This applies particularly to social diagnoses, ten per cent of which received anxiolytics. Also, the increase of these prescriptions with age intensifies this impression, because older people appeared especially likely to suffer from mood disturbances, requiring recognition and discussion, according to Goldberg.

Something positive about prescription should be said regarding patients presenting physical symptoms, considered psychological by the general practitioner. These somatizers received remarkably few psychotropic drugs. As far as anxiolytics and hypnotics are concerned, this is in line with Goldberg's advice. Unfortunately, they hardly received any anti-depressants either, which would have been indicated in a number of cases.

We should also conclude that referral is much more rare than it should be according to psychiatrists. Although the rare cases of psychoses have been referred relatively the most often, as they should have been, the overall referral rate is low.

Older patients and females, in particular, more at risk for psychological diagnoses and presumably also for "disorders that requiring specific interventions" are underrepresented in the referred cases.

Counselling has been recorded extensively. It is difficult to evaluate its appropriateness. One remark can be made about counselling: in cases where a physical diagnosis is paired with a suspicion of a psychological background, exploring the backgrounds of the complaints is found relatively rarely. A lot of psychosocial suspicions seem to remain unspoken. Perhaps this is one of the main differences between the general medical setting of general practice and the psychiatric settings.

And finally, a narrow look at the management of psychosocial diagnoses brings us back at our point of departure: patients requests. For, the management of mental disorder seems dependent upon a psychological or social complaint. When a psychosocial diagnosis is based on physical complaints, the probability of a psychiatric kind of management of the problem (an active kind of counselling, psychopharmacological therapy or mental health referral) has already been drastically reduced. This is even more the case when the general practitioner considers physical diagnoses partly psychological by nature. It does not make much difference if these patients are subjectively or objectively in need.

Although viewed from "general practitioner-friendly" - criteria, treatment of psychological disorder shows a lot of shortcomings. The possible psychological background of physical complaints is not discussed in most cases, too many patients are kept happy with repeat prescriptions, not much attention is paid to possible alternative ways of coping with stressful circumstances and it remains to be seen how many patients whose disorders require specific interventions are overlooked. The hard assignment for the general practitioner is to attune his treatment to the demands of the patient and to estimate the alternatives and other resources the patient may have to deal with his problems. From that perspective it is feasible that, contrary to Goldberg's advice, a general practitioner keeps handing over the repeat prescriptions for sleeping pills to the old lady, requiring support and social intervention. If alternatives are hard to find, support has to be given by meeting the patient's demands. But it is to be recommended that these situations become more exceptions than the rule[1]. Rules about proper prescription. Rules about the diagnosis of depression. Rules that should be taught general practitioners. In the Netherlands vocational training of general practitioners was introduced as a 1-year program in the early seventies, it was extended to two years some years ago and it is to become a 3-year program. It is essential that psychiatry departments contribute significantly to this curriculum. This contribution should not be made in the clinics but in ambulatory settings and if possible in general practice settings.

Consultation by liaison psychiatrists, already briefly mentioned in the section on the "primacy of demand", is another opportunity to inform general practitioners about therapeutic possibilities.

However, the delicate balance between doctor's insights and patient's wishes requires not only cognitive and treatment skills from the general practitioner, but, above all, an excellent mastery of the process of interaction with the patient. The general practitioner has been pictured repeatedly as a mediator between patient's demand and his needs, as established by psychiatrists. The general practitioner should depart from the subjective need of the patient, should take his request very seriously but he may need to add something to it. On the other hand, he should have the psychiatric classification as a guideline in mind, in order not to miss important psychiatric disorders (Goldberg's third category). Given the specific characteristics of a primary care population, he will usually not arrive at neat psychiatric DSM-III diagnoses, but at a range from normal to abnormal on a number of dimensions. Symptom diagnoses will be his part.

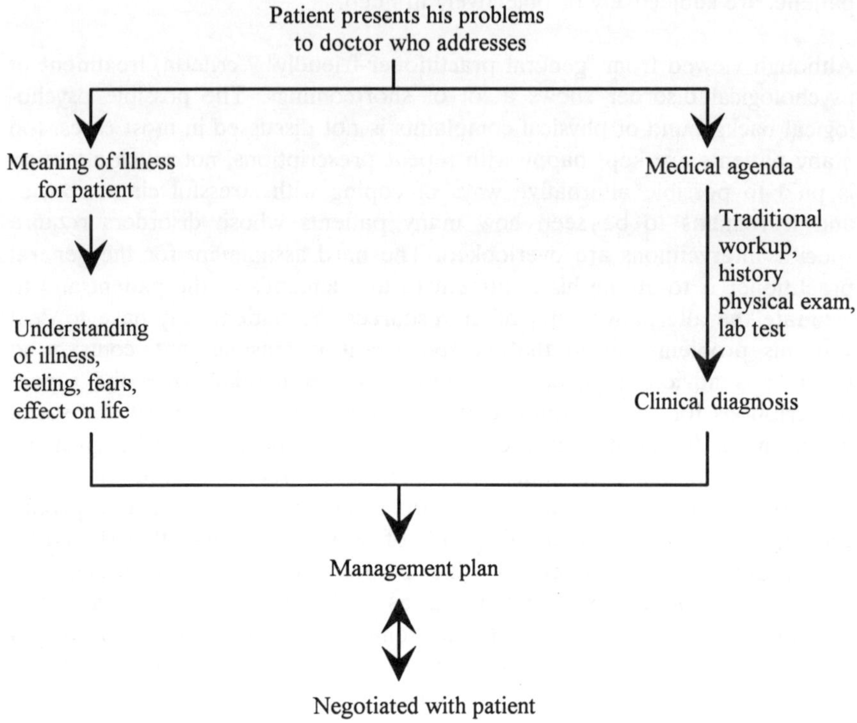

Figure 6.1 The patient-centered clinical method

McWhinney and colleagues developed a model for doctor-patient interaction which may serve to bridge the gap between patient's demand and needs according to the psychiatrist (McWhinney 1989).

At first the reason for visit must be established. During this introductory phase facilitating, patient-centered behaviour is recommended (See the recommendations on recognition, above. Cf. also Goldberg 1979). Next comes the history. Essentially in the model there are the two parallel tracks the general practitioner must keep in mind: the meaning of illness for the patient (patient demands) and the medical agenda (which in this case leans heavily on the psychiatric diagnostic models, but the biomedical aspect should not be neglected, for instance in case of somatization). This is the phase in which the general practitioner might feel obliged to depart from the patient demands, for instance because of lack of objective evidence for his physical complaints. This is on the other hand also the phase in which the general practitioner may suspect an anxiety disorder, but will choose to stick to the demand of the patient to help him with his sleeping problems.

Considerations about patient's supporting power, his reason for a visit at this particular time, and knowledge about patient's coping style in general will play an important role in the decision making process.

This two-track history may end with an agreement between doctor and patient about the nature of the complaints and a management plan.

When we consider our results within the light of this model, it may explain why the general practitioner has more psychosocial assessments than psychological or social complaints, on the one hand, while a number of patients with psychiatric needs according to psychiatrists remain undiagnosed. Therefore, a very important skill, the general practitioner should add to his communicative repertoire is the explicit discussion of his assumptions about the psychosocial character of the symptoms presented. It may prove a hard assignment and more research will be needed to develop fruitful models, but it seems a necessary condition to break through the vicious circle of non-demand → recognition → non-treatment.

The General Practitioner should end up higher than patient's demand, but not necessarily at the level of psychiatric assessment: it is most important to develop those diagnostic skills to such an extent that a general practitioner can make a reasonable interpretation of the patients complaints from a psychiatric perspective. It is still more important, I believe, for a general practitioner to develop an interaction style that makes him really competent to assess the meaning of illness for the patient, and thus to act in conformity to his wishes without denying his clinical diagnosis.
Not so much "let the patient's wish be the doctor's command", but "let doctors incorporate patient's demand in their own view".

The last word directed to the patient: mental health education

Patients could relieve general practitioners' assignment to incorporate patient's demands into their views enormously. In particular that group with disorders, requiring specific interventions, who choose not to discuss their problems with the general practitioner, while they would benefit from such discussion if they did. Bensing and Verhaak (1994) have suggested that the problem could as well be laid with the patient. Departing from the opinion that the initiative for requiring psychological help should be placed with the patient, the public should be informed more systematically about the undesirability of translating feelings of psychological unwell-being into physical complaints. Health education has changed smoking behaviour, cholesterol intake and jogging habits, why should it not change the interpretation of unspecified bodily sensations? In the same spirit, Jenkins (1992) pleads for "universal measures eg educating children and adolescents:

> Children and adolescents need to develop a core of stored knowledge and basic understanding about physical and psychological development and personal needs... It is also important to help them develop constructive attitudes towards mental illness - including its treatability and to understand the need to combat stigma. Such knowledge can help young people pass from childhood dependence to adult life more successfully; (Jenkins 1992, p.14).

The idea is attractive but must be accompanied by some caveats.
The most important one has been running like a thread through our argument: many psychological problems cannot simply be cured. It would be unwise to convince people that there is an answer to all their questions when help is not available. It would be wise to put mental health education to the same tests as other preventive measures: the underlying mechanism should be known and demonstrated and the preventive measure should not cause many "false positives" demanding help unnecessarily.

A second warning follows naturally from the first: in order to avoid somatization, massive "psycholigization" is not to be recommended.

Mental health education should be directed at "de-stigmatization" of requesting psychological help, it should be directed at those groups at risk for which suitable treatment is available, and it should leave the initiative to the patients: "bring your demand into the view of the doctor!"

In this way, all parties involved, patient, general practitioner and psychiatric epidemiology may contribute to closing the gap between doctor's views and patient's demands.

Notes

1. Recently the Dutch College of General Practitioners published a standard on depression. In case of severe depression (= DSM-IIIR "major depression" counseling, possibly in combination with anti-depressants prescription is recommended. Follow-up appointments are strongly advised. In case of mild depression anti-depressants are not considered very worthwhile. Follow-up is restricted to the cases where symptoms worsen in course of time.

Literature

American Psychiatric Association (1980), *Diagnostic and Statistical Manual, 3thd edition*, APA, Washington.

Andersen R., Newman JF., (1973) Societal and individual determinants of Medical Care Utilization in the United Stated. *Millbank Memorial Fund Quarterly*, 51, pp. 95-124.

Angst J. (1990), *Depression and anxiety: a review of studies in the community and in primary care*, In: Sartorius, N., Goldberg, D., Girolamo G. de, et al (eds), Psychological disorders in general medical settings, pp. 60-68, Hogrefe & Huber, Toronto.

Arindell, W.A., and Ettema, J.H.M. (1986), *SCL-90. Handleiding bij een multidimensionele psychopathologie-indicator.* Swets Test Services, Lisse.

Bauduin, D. (ed) (1988), *A Guide to Mental Health Care in the Netherlands.* NcGv, Utrecht.

Bellantuono, C., Fiorio, R., Zanotelli, R. and Tansella, M. (1987), Psychiatric screening in general practice in Italy, *Social Psychiatry*, 22, pp. 113-117.

Bensing, J.M. (1991a), *Doctor-patient communication and the quality of care,* Dissertation, Rotterdam.

Bensing, J.M. (1991b), Doctor-patient communication and the quality of care, *Social Science and Medicine*, Vol. 32, No. 11, pp. 1301-1310.

Bensing, J.M. (1992), Instrumental and affective aspects of doctor-patient communication, *Medical Care*, Vol. 30, No. 4, pp.283-298

Bensing, J.M. (1994), *De rotonde van lichaam en geest*, Inaugural adress Utrecht University.

Bensing, J.M. and Beerendonk, Ph.M. (1990), Psychosociale problemen in de huisartspraktijk: weten en meten, *Maandblad Geestelijke Volksgezondheid*, 45, pp. 595-618.

Bensing, J.M. and Verhaak, P.F.M. (1994), Psychische problematiek in de huisartspraktijk, een generalistisch perspectief, *Nederlands Tijdschrift voor Geneeskunde*, 138, 3, pp. 130-135.

Berne, E. (1964), Games people play. Penguin books, Harmondsworth.

Boerma, W.G.W., Jong, F.A.J.M. de, and Mulder, P.H. (1993), *Health care and general practice across Europe*, NIVEL/NHG, Utrecht.

Bradburn, N.M. (1969), *The structure of psychological well-being*, Aldine, Chicago.

Bridges, K., Goldberg, D., Evans B. and Sharpe, T. (1991), Determinants of somatization in primary care. *Psychological Medicine*, 21, pp. 473-483.

Buitink, J. (1993), *Op één lijn. De hulpvraag, hulpverlening, organisatie, kwaliteit, imago een toekomst van het Algemeen Maatschappelijk Werk in Nederland*, SWP, Utrecht.

Collijn, D., Wijkel D., Feltz-Cornelis, C.M. van der, Verhaak, P.F.M. and Huyse F.J. (1994), *Psychiatrische consulten bij somatiserende patiënten in de huisartspraktijk*, NIVEL/VU, Utrecht/Amsterdam.

Crombie, D.L. (1963), The procrustean bed of medical nomenclature, *The Lancet*, June 1, pp. 1205-1206.

Crombie, D.L. and Zee, J. van der (1982), *The feasibility of a national general practice morbidity and intervention survey in the Netherlands; report of a symposium*, NIVEL, Utrecht.

DeMarco, R. (1984), Relationship between physical and psychological symptomatology in the 22-item Langner's scale, *Social Science and Medicine*, 19, 1, pp. 59-65.

Derogatis, L.R. (1977), *SCL-90R (revised) Manual I. Clinical Psychometrics Research Unit*, Johns Hopkins University School of Medicine, Baltimore.

Deyo, R.A., Inui, T.S., Leininger, J.D., et al. (1983), Measuring functional outcomes in chronic disease: a comparaison of traditional scales and a self-administered health status questionnaire in patients with reumathoid arthritis, *Medical Care* 21, 180-192.

Dohrenwend, B.P. (1990), 'The problem of validity in field studies of psychological disorders' revisited. *Psychological Medicine*, 20, pp. 195-206

Dohrenwend, B.P., Shrout, P.E., Egri, G. and Mendelsohn F.S., (1980) Non-specific Psychological Distress and other dimensions of psychopathology. *Arch. Gen. Psychiatry*, 37, 11, pp.1229-1236.

Eisenberg, L. (1992), The science of epidemiology: empirical data gathering, public-healh action, or both? In Cooper, B. and Eastwood, R., *Primary health care and psychiatric epidemiology*, Routledge, London

Eysenck, H.J., Wakefield, J.A. and Friedman A.F. (1983), Diagnosis and clinical assessment, the DSM-III. *Ann. Rev. Psychol.*, 34, pp.167-193.

Finlay-Jones, R.A. and Burvill, P.W. (1977), The prevalence of minor psychiatric morbidity in the community, *Psychological Medicine*, 7, pp. 475-489.

Fleming, D.M. and Backer, P. (eds) (1992), *The European study of referrals from primary to secondary care*. RCGP occasional paper 56, Royal College of General Practitioners, London.

Foets, M. and Sixma, H. (1991), *Een Nationale Studie van ziekten en verrichtingen in de huisartspraktijk. Basisrapport: Gezondheid en gezondheidsgedrag in de praktijkpopulatie,* NIVEL, Utrecht.

Foulds, G. (1976), *The hierarchical nature of personal illness,* Academic Press, London.

Friele, R.D. and Verhaak, P.F.M. (1991), *Vragen om problemen: een onderzoek onder de volwassen cliënten van RIAGG en AMW*, NIVEL, Utrecht.

Furer, J.W. and Tax, B. (eds) (1987), *Somatische klachten, psychiatrische symptomen en psychosociale problemen. Eindrapport Regioprojekt Nijmegen, deel 1. Juni 1987* Instituut voor Sociale Geneeskunde, K.U., Nijmegen.

Gater, R., De Almeida e Sousa, B., Barrientos, G., Caraveo, J., Chandrashekar, C.R., Dhadphale, M., Goldberg, D., Al Kathiri, A.H., Mubbashar, M., Silhan Km Thong, D., Torres-Gonzales, F. and Sartorius, N., (1991), The pathways to psychiatric care: a cross-cultural study, *Psychological Medicine*, 21, pp. 761-774.

Giel, R. (1982), *Waarom een psychiatrische diagnose,* Stafleu, Alphen a/d Rijn / Brussel.

Giel, R., Koeter, M.W.J. and Ormel, J. (1990), Detection and referral of Primary Care patients with mental health problems: the second and third filter In: Goldberg D, Tantam D, (eds), *The public health impact of mental disorder.* Hogrefe & Huber, Toronto.

Giel, R., Koeter, M.W.J., Meer, K. vd and Ormel, J. (1991), De filters in het model van Goldberg en Huxley in de praktijk, *Huisarts & Wetenschap*, 34, 4, pp. 169-172.

Goldberg, D.P. (1972), *The detection of psychiatric illness by questionnaire,* Oxford university press, London.

Goldberg, D. (1974), Screening for disease, *The Lancet*, pp. 1245-1247.

Goldberg, D. (1979), Detection and assessment of emotional disorders in a primary care setting. *Int. J. Ment. Health*, 8, 2, pp. 30-48.

Goldberg, D. (1985), Identifying psychiatric illness among general medical patients, *British Medical Journal*, 291, pp. 161-162.

Goldberg, D. (1992), A classification of psychological distress for use in primary care settings, *Social Science & Medicine*, 35, 2, pp. 189-193.

Goldberg, D.P. and Blackwell, B. (1970), Psychiatric illness in general practice. A detailed study using a new method of case identification, *British Medical Journal*, 2, pp. 439-443.

Goldberg, D., Kay, C. and Thompson L. (1976), Psychiatric morbidity in general practice and the community, *Psychological Medicine*, 6, pp. 565-569.

Goldberg, D. and Huxley, P. (1980), *Mental illness in the community: the pathway to psychiatric care*, Tavistock Publications, London.

Goldberg, D. and Bridges, K. (1987), Screening for psychiatric illness in general practice: the general practitioner versus the screening questionnaire, *Journal of the Royal College of General Practitioners*, 37, 1, pp. 15-18.

Goldberg, D.P., Bridges, K., Duncan-Jones and P., Grayson, D. (1987), Dimensions of neuroses seen in primary care settings. *Psychological Medicine*, 17, pp. 461-470.

Goldberg, D. and Huxley, P. (1992), *Common mental disorderss, a bio-social model*, Tavistock/Routledge, London and New York.

Groot, M.J.W. de (1971), De "geestelijke verzieking" van het Nederlandse volk. *Medisch Contact*, 26, pp. 815-822.

Hafner, H. (1987), The concept of disease in psychiatry, *Psychological Medicine*, 17, pp. 11-14.

Henderson, A.S., Duncan-Jones, P., Byrne, D.G., Scott, R. and Adcock S. (1979), Psychiatric disorder in Canberra: a standardised study of prevalence. *Acta Psychiatrica Scandinavica*, 60, pp. 335-374.

Her Majesty's Stationery Office (1986), *Morbidity Statistics from General Practice. Third National Study 1981-82 (series MB 5, no.1)*, HMSO, London.

Hodiamont, P.P.G. (1983), Het 'wat' in de psychiatrische epidemiologie, *Tijdschrift voor psychiatrie*, 25, 6, pp. 391-405.

Hodiamont, P., Heine, E.J.H. ter, Heydendael, P.H.J.M., Furer, J.W. and Peer, P.G.M. (1986), Psychiatrische en psychosociale problematiek: overeenkomst en verschil: resultaten van een bevolkingsonderzoek in de Nijmegen. *Maandblad Geestelijke Volksgezondheid*, 41, 2, pp. 128-144.

Hodiamont, P., Peer, N. and Syben, N. (1987), Epidemiological aspects of psychiatric disorder in a Dutch health area. *Psychological Medicine*, 17, pp. 495-505.

Hoeper, E.W., Nycz, G.R., Cleary, P.D., Regier, D.A. and Goldberg, I.D. (1979), Estimated prevalence of RDC mental disorder in primary medical care, *International Journal of Mental Health*, 8, 2, pp. 6-15.

Hofmans-Okkes, I.M., Lamberts, H. and Hofmans E.A. (1992), De paradox van de patiëntgerichte benadering. *Huisarts en Wetenschap*, 35, 7, pp. 281-286.

Hunt, S.M., McEwan, J., McKenna, S.P. (1986), *Measuring health status*, Croom Helm, London.

Jencks, S.F. (1985), Recognition of mental distress and diagnosis of mental disorder in primary care, *JAMA*, 253, pp. 1903-1907.

Jenkins, R. (1992), Depression and anxiety: an overview of preventive strategies. In: Jenkins, R., Newton, J., and Young R.,: *The prevention of depression and anxiety*, London, HMSO,

Jenkins, R., Smeeton, N. and Shepherd, M. (1988), Classification of Mental Disorder in Primary Care, *Psychological Medicine*, Supplements, 12.

Jong, G. de, (1986), *Ongelijkheid in gezondheid; Sociaal-medisch onderzoek en beleid*, Disseratie, Rotterdam.

Katon, W., Korff, M., Lin, E., et al. (1990), Distressed high utilizers of medical care DSM-III-R diagnoses and treatment needs. *General Hospital Psychiatry*, 12, pp. 355-362.

Katon, W., Van Korff, M., Lin, E., Bush, T. an Ormel J. (1992), Adequacy and duration of anti-depressant treatment in primary care, *Medical Care*, 30, 1, pp. 67-76.

Kessler, L.G., Amick, III, B.C., Thompson, J. (1985), Factors influencing the diagnosis of mental disorder among primary care patients. *Medical Care*, 23, 1, pp. 50-62.

Kessler, L.G., Burns, B.J., Shapiro, S., Tischler, G.L., George, L.K., Hough, R.L., Bodison, D. and Miller, R.H. (1987), Psychiatric diagnoses of medical service users: evidence from the Epidemiological Catchment Area Program, *American Journal of Public Health*, 77, 1, pp. 18-24.

Klerman, G.L. (1990), Paradigm shiftsin USA psychiatric epidemiology since World War II. *Soc Psychiatry and Psychiatric Epidemiology*, 20, pp. 27-32.

Klerman, G.L., Olfson, M., Leon, A.C. and Weissman, M.M. (1992), Measuring the need for mental health care. *Health Affairs*, Fall 1992, pp. 23-33.

Koeter, M. (1992), *Wat is ons eigen oordeel waard? De vragenlijstmethode in de psychiatrie,* Dissertatie, Groningen.

Koeter, M.W.J., Ormel, J., Brink, W. v.d., Dijkstra, W., Schoenmacker, J. and Staal, J. (1987), De waarde van de GHQ als toestandsmaat. *Tijdschrift voor psychiatrie*, 29, 10, pp. 667-679.

Lamberts, H. (1982), Psychosocial problems and the disease model: two major determinants of primary health care delivery. In: Lipkin, M. and Kupka, K., (eds) *Psychosocial Factors affecting health*. Praeger Publishers, New York.

Lamberts, H. (1991), *In het huis van de huisarts. Verslag van het transitieproject*, MEDI-tekst, Lelystad.

Lamberts, H. and Hartman B. (1982), Psychische en sociale problemen in de huisartspraktijk. *Huisarts & Wetenschap*, 25, pp. 333-342.

Lamberts, H., Meads, S. and Wood M. (1982), *The reason for encounter classification for use in primary care*, Field trial version july 1982.

Lamberts, H. and Wood, M. (eds) (1987), *International Classification of Primary Care*, Oxford University Press, Oxford.

Leaf, P.J. and Bruce, M.L. (1987), Gender differences in the use of mental health-related services: a re-examination, *Journal of Health and Social Behavior*, 28, 2, pp. 171-183.

Lehtinen, V., Joukamaa, M., Jyrkinen, E., Lahtela, K., Raitasalo, R., Maatela, J., Aromaa, A. (1990), Need for mental health services of the adult population in Finland: results from the Mini Finland Health Survey, *Acta Scand. Psych*, 5, pp. 426-431.

Leighton, D. (1956), The distribution of psychiatric symptoms in a small town. *American Journal of Psychiatry*, 112, p. 716.

Limbeek, J. van, Berg, C.E.A. van den, Sergeant, J.A., Geerlings, P.J., Fransman, J.M.L. (red.) (1994), *Patiënt, stoornis en zorg. Een onderzoek naar de prevalentie, het ziektebeloop en de herkenning van psychische stoornissen in Amsterdam Oost en Zuidoost*, GG&GD, Amsterdam.

Lisdonk, E.H. v.d. (1988), *Ervaren en aangeboden morbiditeit in de huisartspraktijk*, Dissertatie, Nijmegen.

Lisdonk, E.H. van de, Bosch, W.J.H.M. van den, Huygen, F.J.A., Lagro-Janssen, A.L.M. (red.) (1990), *Ziekten in de huisartspraktijk*, Wetenschappelijk Uitgeverij Bunge, Utrecht.

Mari, J. and Williams, P. (1986), Misclassification by psychiatric screening questionnaires. *J Cron. Diss.*, 5, pp. 371-378.

Marks, J.N., Goldberg, D.P. and Hillier, V.F. (1979), Determinants of the ability of general practitioners to detect psychiatric illness. *Psychological Medicine*, 9, pp. 337-353.

McGuire, R.J. (1973), Classification and the problem of diagnosis. In: Eysenck, H.J., *Handbook of abnormal psychology*, Pitman and sons, London.

McWhinney, I.R. (1989), *A textbook of Family Medicine*, Oxford University Press, New York.

Mechanic, D. (1986), The concept of illness behaviour: culture, situation and personal predisposition. *Psychological Medicine*, 16, pp. 1-7.

Meer, K.v.d. (1994), *Patiënten met psychische en sociale problemen in de huisartspraktijk*, Proefschrift Groningen. Lelystad, Meditekst.

Myers, J.K., Wasserman, M.M., Tischler, G.L., Holzer, C.E., Leaf, P.J., Orvaschel, H., Anthony, J.C., Boyd, J.H., Burke, J.D., Kramer, M. and Stoltzman, R., (1984), Six-month prevalence of psychiatric disorders in three communities. *Archives of General Psychiatry*, 41, 10, pp. 959-967.

Narrow, W.E., Regier, D.A., Rae, D.S., Manderscheid, R.W. and Locke, B.Z. (1993), Use of services by persons with mental and addictive disorders, *Arch Gen Psychiatry*, 50, 2, pp. 95-107.

Offerhaus, R. (1978), *Van probleem tot psychiatrie.* St Bavo, Noordwijkerhout.

Office of Population Censuses and Surveys / Royal College of General Practitioners (1986), *Morbidity Statistics from General Practice 1981-1982.* Third National Study. HMSO London.

Orleans, C.S., George, L.K., Houpt, J.L. and Brodie, H.K.H. (1985), How primary care physicians treat psychiatric disorders: a National Survey of Family Practitioners, *American Journal of Psychiatry*, 142, 1, pp. 52-57.

Ormel, J. (1980), *Moeite met leven of een moeilijk leven.* Dissertatie Groningen, Konstapel.

Ormel, J., Koeter, M.W.J., Brink, W. v.d. and Giel, R. (1989), Concurrent validity of GHQ-28 en PSE as measures of change, *Psychological Medicine*, 19, pp. 1007-1013.

Ormel, J., Brink, W. v.d., Koeter, M.W.J., Giel, R., Meer, K. v.d., Willige, G. v.d. and Wilmink, F.W. (1990), Recognition, management and outcome of psychological disorders in primary care: a naturalistic follow-up study, *Psychological Medicine*, 20, pp. 909-923.

Ormel, J. and Giel, R. (1990), Medical effects of nonrecognition of affective disorders in primary care. In: *Psychological disorders in general medical settings*. Sartorius, N., Goldberg, D., Girolamo, G., Costa e Silva, J., Lecrubier, Y. and Wittchen, U. (eds). Hogrefe & Huber Publishers, Toronto, pp. 146-158.

Ormel, J., Koeter, M.W.J., Brink, W. v.d., Willige, G. v.d. (1990), The extent of nonrecognition of mental health problems in Primary Care and its effects on management and outcome. In: Goldberg, D. and Tantam, D. (eds), *The public health impact of mental disorder*, Hogrefe & Huber, Toronto.

Ormel, J., Koeter, M.W.J., Brink, W. v.d. and Willige, G. v.d. (1991), Recognition, Management and course of anxiety and depression in general practice, *Archives of General Psychiatry*,48, 8, pp. 700-706.

Radlof, L.S. (1977), The CES-D scale: a self-report depression scale for research in the general population. *Applied Psychological Measurement*, 1, pp. 385-401.

Regier, D., Narrow, W.E., Rae, D.S., Manderscheid, R.W., Locke, B.Z. and Goodwin, F.K. (1993), The de facto US mental and addictive disorders services system. *Arch Gen Psychiatry*, 50, 2, pp. 85-94.

Ridder, D. de (1988), *Determinanten van psychische gezondheid*, NcGv, Utrecht.

Robins, L.N. and Regier, D.A. (eds) (1991), *Psychiatric disorderds in America: the Epidemiological Catchment Area Study*, Free Press, New York.

Scheff, T.J. (1966), *Being mentally ill. A sociological theory*, Aldine Publishing Company. Chicago.

Schulberg, H.C., Saul, M., McClelland, M., Ganguli, M., Christy, W. and Frank, R. (1985), Assessing depression in primary medical and psychiatric practices. *Archives of General Psychiatry*, 42, 12, pp. 1164-1170.

Schulberg, H.C., McClelland, M. and Burns, B. (1987), Depression and physical illness: The prevalence, causation and diagnosis of comorbidity. *Clinical Psychology Review*, 7, pp. 145-167.

Schulberg, H.C. and Burns, B. (1988), Mental disorder in primary caree. Epidemiologic, diagnostic and treatment research directions. *General Hospital Psychiatry*, 10, pp. 79-87.

Schurman, R.A., Kramer, P.D. and Mitchell, J.B. (1985), The hidden mental Health Network, *Archives of general psychiatry*, 42, 1, pp. 89-94.

Shapiro, S., Skinner, E.A., Kessler, L.G., Von Korff, M., German, P.S., Tischler, G.L., Leaf, P.J., Benham, L., Cottler, L., Regier, D.A. (1984), Utilization of health and mental health services. *Archives of General Psychiatry*, 41, 10, pp. 971-978.

Shepherd, M. (1983), Beyond the layman's madness: the extent of mental disease. In: Shepherd, M., *The psychosocial matrix of of psychiatry.* Tavistock, London.

Shorter, E. (1994), *From the mind into the body. The cultural origins of psychosomatic symptoms*. The free Press, New York.

Shrout, P.E., Dohrenwend, B.P. and Levav, I. (1986), A discriminant rule for screening cases of diverse diagnostic types: preliminary results. *Journal of Consulting Clinical Psychology*, 54, pp. 314-319.

Skuse, D. and Williams, P. (1984), Screening for psychiatric disorder in general practice *Psychological Medicine*, 14, pp. 365-377.

Smith, G.R., Manson, R.A. and Ray, D.C. (1986), Psychiatric consultations in somatization disorder, *New England Journal of Medicine*, 314, 22, pp. 1407-1413.

Swaan, A. de (1979), *Sociologie van de psychotherapie,* Spectrum, Utrecht.

Swartling, P.G., Kebbon, L. and Smedby, B. (1987), Mental health problems in primary health care as seen by doctors. *Scand. J. Prim. Health Care*, 5, pp. 201-204.

Taylor, A. and Chave, S. (1964), *Mental health and environment*, Clay & Bungay.

Taylor, F. Kraupl (1971), A logical analysis of the medico-psychological concept of disease. Part 1 and Part 2, *Psychological Medicine*, 1, pp. 356-364\ 2, pp. 7-16.

Terluin, B. (1994), Overspanning onderbouwd (Nervous Breakdown Substatiated). Proefschrift Utrecht.

Trimbos, C.J.B.J. (1971), De "geestelijke verzieking" van het Nederlandse volk. Reactie op M.de Groot, *Medisch Contact*, 26, pp. 981-982.

Vázquez-Barquero, J.L., Diez Manrique, J.F., Pena, C., Aldama, J., Samaniego, C., Menendez Arango, J. and Mirapeix, C. (1987), A community mental health survey in Cantabria, *Psychological Medicine*, 17, pp. 227-241.

Vázquez-Barquero, J.L., Pena, C., Diez Manrique, J.F., Arenal, A., Quinatanal, R.G. and Samaniego, C. (1988), The influence of sociocultural factors on the interaction between physical and mental disturbances in a rural community. *Social Psychiatry and Psychiatric epidemiology*, 23, pp. 195-201.

Vázquez-Barquero, J.L., Wilkinson, G., Williams, P., Diez-Manrique, J.F. and Pena, C. (1990), Mental health and medical consultation in primary care settings, *Psychological Medicine*, 20, pp. 681-694.

Verhaak, P.F.M. (1986), *Interpretatie en behandeling van psychische klachten in de huisartspraktijk* (Interpretation and treatment of psychological complaints in general practice), Dissertatie, Rotterdam.

Verhaak, P.F.M. (1988), Detection of psychological complaints by general practitioners. *Medical Care*, 26, pp. 1009-1020.

Verhaak, P.F.M. (1993), Analysis of referrals of mental health problems by general practitioners, *British Journal of General Practice*, 43, pp. 203-208.

Verhaak, P.F.M. *Mental illness and help-seeking behaviour*, accepted by Psychological Medicine.

Verhaak, P.F.M. and Wennink, H.J. (1990), What does a doctor do with psychosocial complaints in primary care. *Int.J.Psychiatry in Medicine*, 20, 2, pp. 151-162.

Verhaak, P.F.M., Wennink, H.J. and Tijhuis, M.A.R. (1990), The importance of the GHQ in general practice. *Family Practice*, 7, pp. 319-324.

Verhaak, P.F.M. and Tijhuis, M.A.R. (1994), The Somatizing patient in primary care, *International Journal of Psychiatry in Medicine*, 24, 2, pp. 163-183.

Verhey, R., Bakker, D.H. de, and Velden, J. van der (1992), *De huisarts in de grote stad*. NIVEL, Utrecht.

White, K.L. (1988), *The task of medicine*. Dialogue at Wickenburg. Henry Kaiser Family Foundation, Menlo Park, California.

Wiegersma, Tj. and Meulenberg, F. (1993), Consultvoering, quo vadis? *Huisarts en Wetenschap*, 36, 6/7, pp. 223-226.

Wilkinson, M.J.B. and Barczak, P. (1988), Psychiatric screening in general practice: comparison of the general health questionnaire and the hospital anxiety scale. *Journal of Royal College of General Practitioners*, 38, 7, pp. 311-313.

Wilkinson, G. and Markus, A.C. (1989), Validation of a computerized assessment (PROQSY) of minor psychological morbidity by Relative Operating Characteristic analysis using a single GP's assessment as criterion measures, *Psychological Medicine*, 19, pp. 225-231.

Williams, P., Tarnapolsky, A., Hand, D. and Shepher, M. (1986), Minor psychiatric morbidity and general practice consultations: the West London Survey, *Psychological Medicine Monograph*, Supplement 9.

Wilmink, F.M. (1989), *Patient, physician, psychiatrist. Assessment of mental health problems in primary care*, Dissertation Groningen.

Wing, J.K., Mann, S.A., Leff, J.P. and Nixon, J.M. (1978), The concept of a 'case' in psychiatric population surveys. *Psychological Medicine*, 8, pp. 203-217.

Wright, A.F. and Perini, A.F. (1987), Hidden psychiatric illness: use of the general health questionnaire in general practice, *Journal of the Royal College of General Practitioners*, 37, 4, pp. 164-167.

Wright, A.F. (1990), A study of the presentation of somatic symptoms in general practice by patients with psychiatric disturbance. *British Journal of General Practice*, 40, pp. 459-463.

Wulff, H.R., Pederson, S.A. and Rosenberg, R. (1986), Philosophy of medicine. An introduction. Blackwell Scientific Publications, Oxford.

Ypema, E. and Haen, F. de (1983), *Verdelen naar behoefte*, NcGv, Utrecht.

Zee., J.v.d. (1982), *De vraag naar diensten van de huisarts*, Proefschrift Maastricht. Utrecht, NHI.